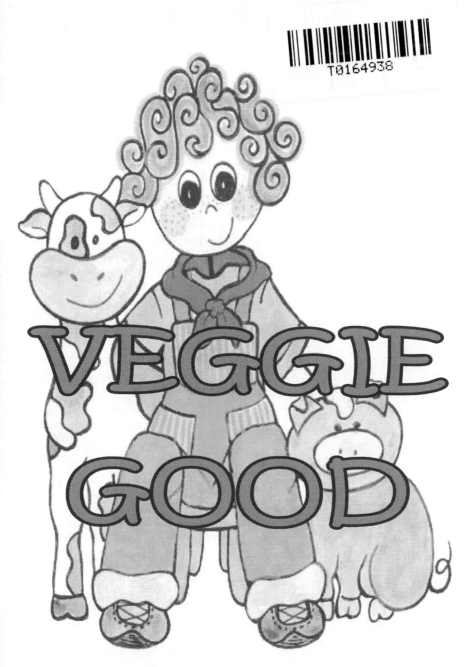

# VEGGIE GOOD

## ANIMALS ARE MY FRIENDS

*Trafford rev. 09/13/2011*

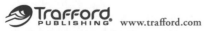 www.trafford.com

North America & international
toll-free: 1 888 232 4444 (USA & Canada)
phone: 250 383 6864 ♦ fax: 812 355 4082

Richie, I could not have done this without your help and
support, thank you.

My dear family, thank you.

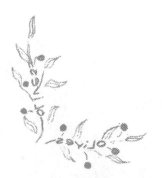
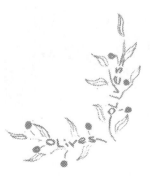

# THE STORY

Roughly 16 years ago everyone in my household decided to be a vegetarian, except me. Seeing as how I am the main cook in this household I had to adapt. This is kind of ironic since I really love animals, go figure. As was to be expected I soon realized that I too, wanted to be a vegetarian.

This book started about 12 years ago when one of my sons decided to make a cookbook for his graduation project in graphic design. He finished his project but I only got as far as jotting down the recipes, with the help of a friend, into a rough draft. Days went by and my idea of writing a vegetarian cookbook, literally, got shoved into a drawer waiting to resurface. Now, with some gentle nudging from my other son; well maybe not so gentle, here I am. Who says mom's don't listen to their children!

There are, of course, different reasons for becoming a vegetarian, religious, humanitarian and health. There are also different types of vegetarians. There are vegans that do not eat any animal by-products like honey, eggs, cheese, milk, yoghurt and of course the obvious, meat, fish, poultry, etc. Then you have ovo- vegetarians that eat eggs, ovo-lacto-vegetarian that eat eggs and milk products, lacto-vegetarian that eat milk products and api-vegetarian that eat honey. Sounds confusing but I'm sure you catch the drift.

By the way, do not think that being a vegetarian is synonymous of losing weight. There are quite a few chubby vegetarians out there. We can eat carbs and sweets and yummy desserts. So, to lose weight you still have to watch what you eat. Sooorryyyy

Many people become vegetarians with no real convictions and soon become discouraged. This happens all the time, specially, because they become bored with the same old same old. They have it "sooooo wrong". Why, you ask? Well for starters you can still have your favorite recipes and simply eliminate the meat part. For instance, my sister makes a delicious " lamb-less" Irish stew, I make a pretty good "chicken-less" pie, one of my sons makes a yummy "chicken-less "ajiaco". Now, my other son made us a super artichoke and spinach lasagna, my sister in-law made us an exotic chicken-less "tagine", and my hubby makes a " killer" meatless tomato salsa for pasta dishes and so on and so forth. You can also buy "veggie" cookbooks like this one to get good ideas or look for recipes on the internet. Once you are on a roll, just let your imagination lead the way. Don't be disheartened by the occasional "flop", it happens to us all. Like the proverbial metaphor, you must get back on the horse right away.

My strongest recommendation to all who read this is book is, "HAVE FUN COOKING". Cooking is an everyday chore for most of us. All the cooking and washing up and grocery shopping can become monotonous and "boring". By trying new recipes, new seasonings, being creative and making new twists and turns with your cooking, you can breathe new life into this daily task making it, guess what? SOMETHING YOU ENJOY.

Another question that people ask themselves is "are you getting the required vitamins, minerals, proteins etc. that your body needs to thrive?" My answer is, of course you must eat a balanced diet with all its requirements which goes the same for when you are not a vegetarian. Proteins are actually in a lot of the things we eat like milk in all of its variations, dried beans, TVP and other soy based foods and gluten in all of

Rosemary

its presentations. Your veggies also supply you with vitamins, minerals and fiber. Never forget to eat plenty of fruit. I feel that even though you are eating a balanced diet you should consult with your family doctor on what vitamin supplements you should take. I personally would recommend that non vegetarians to do the same. Here is a list, of some of the vitamins we require and where it is said you can get them.

Vitamin E – found in mustard greens, turnip greens, chard, sunflower seeds, collard greens, parsley, papaya, olives, Bell peppers, Brussels sprouts, kiwi, tomatoes, blueberries, broccoli, wheat germ, whole grains and nuts.

Beta Carotene: found in carrots, spinach, pumpkin, apricots, peaches, melon and cherries.

Vitamin C: found in red berries, kiwi, red and green bell peppers, tomatoes, broccoli, spinach, guava, grapefruit and oranges.

Vitamin A: found in carrots, sweet potato, pumpkin, spinach, collards and kale.

Q10: found in soybeans, peanuts, sesame seeds, pistachios, walnuts, azuki beans, hazel nuts, almonds, chestnuts, spinach, broccoli, sweet potatoes, sweet peppers, garlic, peas, cauliflower and carrots.

Zinc: found in milk, cheese, yeast, peanuts, whole grain cereals, brown rice, whole wheat bread, potato, yogurt and pumpkin seeds.

Niacin (B3): found in fortified cereals and peanuts.

Vitamin B12: found in milk, cheese, eggs and added to some breakfast cereals.

Vitamin B6: found in Brussels sprouts, collard greens, spinach, bell peppers, turnip greens, garlic, cauliflower, mustard greens, asparagus, broccoli, summer squash, eggplant, onions, green beans, sweet potato, carrots, tomato, leeks, romaine lettuce, avocado, strawberries, watermelon and banana.

Vitamin D: egg yolks and fortified milk.

Omega-3: flax seed

Nevertheless, as I mentioned previously, vegetarians and meat eaters alike should consult their family doctor. By the way, remember you can get your Omega-3 requirements from flax seed. See the "before you start cooking" section for instructions on how to prepare flax seed.

I realize that some of the recipes are big. This is because many of them were developed before my sons married and flew the coop. My boys (hubby and two sons) are very big eaters and so were the friends they invited to join us for many a meal. So feel free to cut them down proportionally to your needs.

After all is said and done, even if you are not a vegetarian but just a veggie fan you can still enjoy these recipes, don't you think?

Rosemary

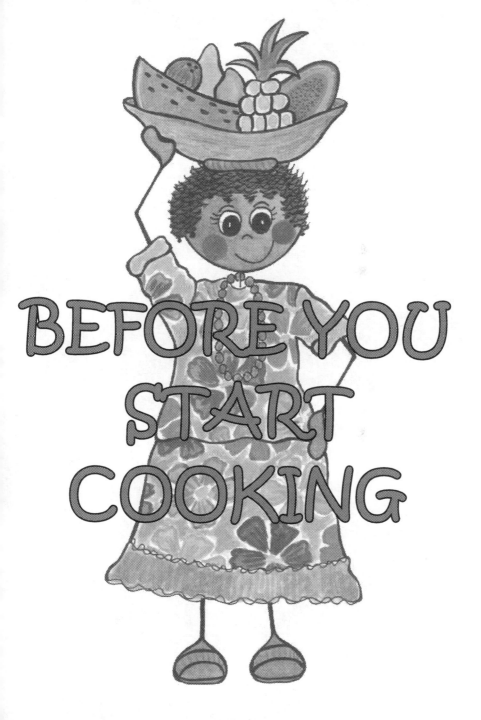

BEFORE YOU START COOKING

## ABREVIATIONS IN THIS BOOK

When you see the letters Tsp. they stand for teaspoon and when you see the letters Tbsp. they stand for tablespoon. You have probably figured this out but just thought I would explain anyway. Do not be confused with TVP (textured vegetable protein) and TSP (textured soy protein).

## PREHEATING OVEN

Remember to preheat your oven 15 to 20 minutes before you start cooking to make sure your oven reaches the required temperature.

## FRESH OR FROZEN VEGETABLES? (WHAT IS BEST)

Really fresh veggies are the best but hey that is not always possible. Don't worry, it is said that canned or frozen produce retain more vitamins since they are processed shortly after being harvested rather than sit in the supermarket for days before being purchased. So take heart. However, if using canned vegetables, read label for sodium content and preservatives.

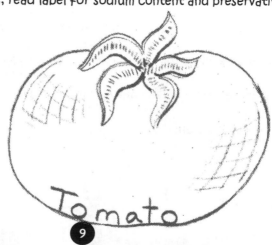

## DO NOT OVERCOOK YOUR PASTA

Cook your pasta "al dente" which means, simply put, do not overcook. It should require a little effort to bite into as opposed to being, "mushy". Anyway, it is said to be less fattening this way.

## WASH YOUR VEGGIES

Please, please, please, make it a habit to wash your veggies before using them. This will eliminate any pesky little bugs or pesticides that may be keeping your veggies company. I can guarantee you will be healthier without them.

## SPINACH

Guess what, spinach contains trace amounts of arsenic which over time accumulates in your system. These easy steps will get rid of this unwanted ingredient. Before you prepare it, wash with abundant water till squeaky clean, place in a colander and pour hot water over it and drain. If you are going to prepare the spinach for a salad, submerge the spinach in a bowl of icy water immediately after pouring the hot water over it. This will stop the cooking process and keep it crunchy.

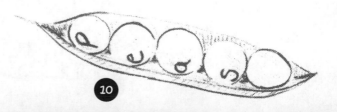

## TOMATOES

If you are using fresh tomatoes, make a small cross-like incision in the bottom of the tomatoes, place in a bowl and cover with boiling water. Leave them covered for about 3 minutes or until you notice that the skin is loose. Discard water, peel and cut the tomatoes and remove the skin and the seeds. Gently squeeze out the water in the tomato. **You are probably asking why go to all this trouble.** This is why. Tomato skins are hard to digest, the water in the tomato can cause acidity and the seeds can get stuck in your digestive tract. I believe it is worth the effort don't you? For salads, just peel them with a potato peeler, cut them in half, remove the seeds and allow to drain for a while.

## BELL PEPPERS

Bell peppers are delicious raw but for many recipes they are even better roasted and **for those who have trouble digesting the peppers they are easier to digest when roasted.** There are different ways, one of which (my favorite) is to place the pepper over a flame rotating slowly, charring the outer skin. Once charred on one side rotate to next position. (Do not over char) Once it is all black (one might think that is beyond repair, but it is ok) then place in a plastic bag or in a covered pot and leave until it is cool to the touch. Proceed to remove the charred skin, the seeds and the stem. Using a spoon to scrape the pimento is one easy way to remove the skin and the seeds. If you add a little olive oil and crushed garlic to the peppers and store them in a sealed container in the refrigerator they will keep for couple of days till ready to be used.

# ARTICHOKES

Artichokes are cooked in a lot of water with a bit of salt for about half an hour. Remove the outer leaves which by the way are delish. Hold the pointy end of the leaf with your fingers scraping off the meaty bottom part of the leaf with your teeth. This is even better if you first dip it in some melted butter with lemon. Mmmmm good! After you have removed the leaves you will encounter a circular cap of fine little hairs. Do not eat this part. Remove these with a small spoon. Now you have an indentation where the hairs were. You have now made contact with the heart of the artichoke. Use them in salads, soups or wherever your imagination leads you.

# EGGPLANT

Eggplant has a tendency to be a tad bitter but you can prevent this by slicing or cubing the eggplant and placing it in a bowl of cold salted water for a half an hour. Remove the salted water, rinse and dry before using.

# COCONUT

Here is a good trick if you are using the coconut "au natural ". Place the coconut over a gas burner and turn slowly on all sides for two or three minutes. It will get a little charred but not blackened. Crack the nut and with a spoon (do not use a knife) loosen the meat from the shell. Heating the outer part of the coconut loosens the white meat inside and it is therefore easier to separate from the shell

# PEPPPER CORNS

Pepper corns (any color) are best used  whole (un-ground), grinding them only when needed to preserve the flavor and freshness.   If you do not have a pepper mill (I must agree with my sister in law when she says that you should fork out for a good one because the cheaper ones just don't do the job and if they do they give out quickly), then you can also use a mortar and pestle or an electric coffee grinder.

## TSP (TEXTURED SOY PROTEIN) OR TVP (TEXTURED VEGETABLE PROTEIN)

TSP (textured soy protein) or TVP (textured vegetable protein) is made from soy. It is usually dehydrated and should be hydrated before using. First you pour hot water over the portion you are going to use and soak for a couple of minutes. Strain the soy meat in a colander and rinse with more hot water. This process eliminates the strong soy flavor which can be somewhat overpowering and unpleasant.

## GLUTEN

Gluten is made from wheat protein and due to its solid consistency can replace meat in any recipe. Gluten can, for some people, be a little heavy on the digestion. It is probably best to have it in small quantities thus avoiding any discomfort. See " Tid Bits Of Information" for gluten recipe.

## TOFU

Tofu is made from soy bean. Comes in its solid presentation resembling cheese or creamy. It is very nutritious and healthy for you. It is used a lot in Asian cooking and it is very versatile. See "Tid Bits of Information" for Tofu recipe.

## SOY CHAFF (BAGASSE)

Soy chaff or "bagasse". If you make soy milk or tofu (see Tid Bits of Information) the leftover chaff can be recycled in soups, veggie hamburgers and stir fries. It still has nutrients and provides fiber.

## THICKENING SOUPS AND SAUCES

There are different ways of thickening soups and sauces. The best way is to make a béchamel or white sauce. The following, is not very professional but it is an easy way: Mix your cornstarch/flour with a small amount of your liquid, dissolving any lumps. When the soup or the sauce is ready, take it off the flame, add the cornstarch/flour mixture stirring well, then return to the burner and simmer till the sauce thickens. I confess that my sons do not agree with this lazy attitude but it works for me and it is quick.

## EGG SUBSTITUTE

In my recipes for cakes I do not use eggs. This is because my husband decided one day that eggs were no longer in his diet so I had to adapt fast. At first I substituted eggs for vinegar, which works fine, but later a friend of mine said she got better results with yoghurt and guess what, she was right. This said, in a pinch, either will do, ok. I replace 1 egg with ¼ C yoghurt or 1 Tbsp vinegar. Replace 2 eggs with 2 Tbsp of vinegar or ½ a cup of yoghurt. Replacing 3 eggs is a little trickier.

## GARLIC

Garlic is said to be beneficial to our health. If you crush it first it is said we benefit even more. I use a mortar and pestle but there are several ways to go about it. Your call.

## BAY LEAF

If using whole leaves always remove before serving. Bay leaves do not soften so the edges can be harmful if eaten.

## COFFEE GRINDER

Coffee grinders are really great to have not only for grinding coffee. In case you haven't heard you can grind whole spices or pepper corns in the coffee grinder. The coffee grinder will keep the fragrance of the spices so you will need a second grinder just for your coffee.

## FLAX SEED

A coffee grinder is great for grinding flax seed. Flax seed should be ground no more than four hours before using otherwise it oxidizes and loses its beneficial properties. Flax seed could cause allergies. It is said that you should start with ¼ teaspoon and work up to 2 tablespoons, stirred in a glass of water or juice. Flax seed is very high in fiber so it may act as a mild laxative and it is a digestive tract cleanser. If you do not have a coffee grinder you can soak the whole flax seed overnight, in a glass of water, and blend before drinking. It is always good idea to consult with your family doctor before trying out something you are not familiar with.

## EXTRA VIRGIN OLIVE OIL

It is said that it is good to use extra virgin olive oil because it is cold pressed, monounsaturated, a source of omega 9 and of course, delish.

## COLD PRESSED GRAPE SEED OIL

I like to use cold pressed grape seed oil because it has a neutral taste. Grape seed oil could cause allergies.

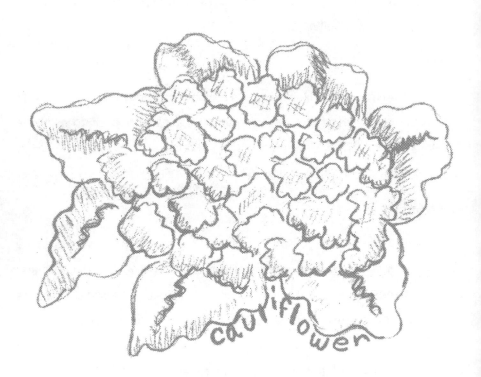

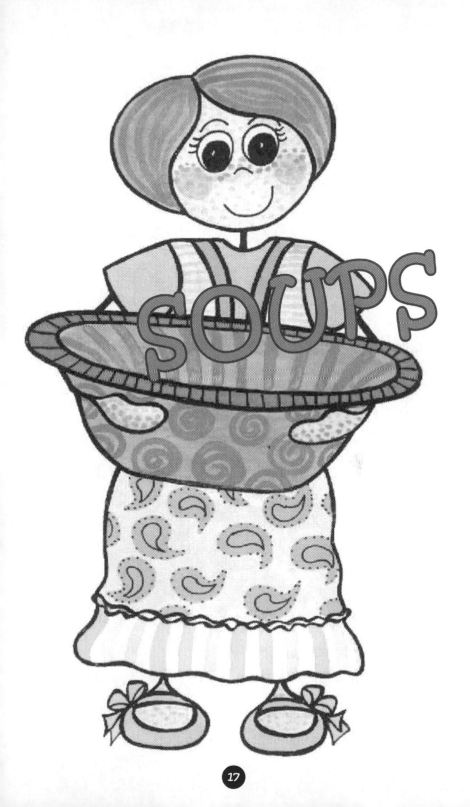

# MUSHROOM **MINESTRONE**

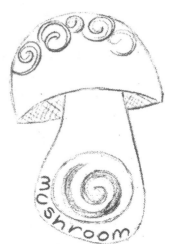

1 Lb. of mushrooms
½ Lb. of onions
1 ½ Lbs. of tomatoes (skinned and seeded)
2 Cups of peas (not dried) fresh or frozen
1 Cup of fresh basil
4 bay leaves
5 Cloves of garlic (pureed)
6 Cups of water
Salt and pepper to taste

Slice the (washed) mushrooms and finely dice the tomatoes and the onions. Finely chop the basil. In a relatively large pot, add the water and all the ingredients except the basil. Cover and boil till the ingredients are cooked. Add the basil. Remove the bay leaf before serving. Enjoy.

# VEGGIE "AJIACO"

This thick potato soup originates in Bogota, Colombia. Traditionally it is made with chicken. The Ingredients can be found in a "latin" supermarket.

3 ½ quarts of water
2 large white or yellow onions
1 ½ Cups of peas frozen or fresh (not dried)
2 Lbs. of potatoes for mashing (floury)
2 Lbs. potatoes (the ones you use for potato salad)
2 Lbs. of "Criollo potatoes" (small, round, floury, yellow potatoes) They grow in Colombia S.A.
2 Cups of whole kernel corn (preferably fresh)
1½ Cups of chopped fresh "guascas" (a leafy Colombian herb)
1 Cup of cream
½ Cup of capers

The "criollo" potatoes should be peeled and cut in half. The other potatoes should be peeled and sliced thickly. If the peas and the corn are fresh, they should cook first till tender then add all the remaining ingredients. Boil till all the ingredients are cooked. If the peas and the corn are frozen then add everything together. The "criollo" potato will disintegrate and make the soup creamy and yellow. Add salt and pepper to taste. The cream and capers are to be added by each person.

## VEGGIE GUMBO

1 Lb. of tomatoes peeled and seeded

1 can of coconut cream

2 Medium size carrots
2 leeks
2 Medium size white onions
2 Chayotes (also known as a vegetable pear)
1 ½ Lbs. of a floury potato
1 Lb. of speckled red beans, cooked and strained
10 Cups of water

Peel and dice the carrots and the chayote. Cut the white part of the leeks in slices. In a large pot add the water, the carrots, the leeks, the chayote, the potato and the coconut milk. When the vegetables are tender, add the beans. Let simmer at medium heat for about 5 minutes. While the soup is simmering make a Salsa or "guiso". Dice the white or yellow onion in a little olive oil till tender. Add the diced tomato and sauté, with salt and pepper, for two or three minutes. Stir into the soup. Serve nice and hot with rice or just by itself.

## ONION SOUP

5 White or yellow medium size onions
6 slices of whole wheat bread
3 Cups of milk
6 Cups of water
Salt and black ground pepper to taste

Grape seed oil or Extra virgin olive oil

Slice the onions and sauté with olive oil till tender. Blend the bread and the milk in a blender till creamy. Mix the sautéed onion, the creamed bread and milk and the water. Salt and pepper to taste. Simmer for about 4 minutes. Soup should be creamy. Serve hot.

## CREAM OF CARROT AND CORN SOUP

1 ½ Cups whole corn kernels (Use frozen corn only in an emergency)
3 carrots
1 Cup of cream (optional)
3 Cups of milk
1 tsp of sugar
5 Cups of water
Salt and freshly ground black pepper

Peel and slice the carrots. In a large pot add the water, carrots, corn, salt and pepper. Cover and boil for 20 minutes. In the blender, blend the carrot and the corn with some of the hot water, the cream and the milk. Return ingredients to the pot and add remaining hot water. If mixture is too thick add a bit more milk. Serve hot

## CREAM OF CAULIFLOWER, PEAS AND ONION SOUP

2 ½ Cups of peas (if you are using fresh peas cook first)
1 large cauliflower cut into bite size pieces
2 green bell peppers, diced
20 pearl onions (peeled)
6 Cups of water

4 Cups of milk
1 ½ tsp. salt
2 tsp. of sugar
2 Tbsp. of cornstarch
2 Tbsp. of flour
Salt and freshly ground green pepper corns
2 Tbsp. of soy sauce

In a large pot add the water, the pearl onions and ground green pepper. Boil for 10 minutes. Add green Bell peppers, cauliflower, sugar, salt and soy sauce and cook for 5 more minutes. Stir the flour and the cornstarch together and blend with a little of the milk. Add the milk and cornstarch mixture and the rest of the milk to the pot. Simmer over medium heat till mixture thickens. Serve hot.

P.S. The secret to this soup is the freshly ground green pepper corns so add as much of it as you want. Keep tasting so that it does not get so spicy that you cannot eat it.

## POTATO CHOWDER

2 ½ Liters of water (10 Cups)
6 large potatoes
3 large white onions
2 ½ Cups of whole kernel corn (preferably fresh but frozen will do)
2 Tbsp. fresh chopped dill or 1 Tbsp. dried dill
1 Lb. Spanish style white cheese, (not mozzarella)
Salt and ground black pepper to taste

Peel and slice the potatoes. Peel and dice the onions. In a large pot add the water, the potatoes, the onions, the corn, the dill and the salt and pepper. Cover the pot and boil till all the ingredients are cooked and the soup thickens. Add the cheese and wait 5 minutes before serving

## CELERY AND TOMATO STEW (good for when you are on a diet)

1 head of celery minus the leaves
8 large tomatoes peeled, seeded (see Before You Start Cooking) and roughly chopped
3 cloves of garlic pureed (more is better)
¼ Cup chopped onion
3 tbsp soy sauce
2 tsp of the seasoning of your choice, Italian or French
½ tsp turmeric powder, optional
Salt and freshly ground black pepper to taste
5 Cups water
2 Cups diced Spanish style white cheese

Put the 5 cups of water in a large pot and add the celery cut into bite size pieces. Add the salt, pepper, turmeric, pureed garlic, onion, soy sauce and your seasoning of choice. Boil for about 3 minutes just so that the celery gets a head start. Add the tomato and simmer for a couple of minutes. Add the cheese all at once and simmer for another couple of minutes. When we are in our "diet mode" we keep the soup in the fridge (it will keep for a couple of days) and have it for both lunch and dinner. Make sure that you cool the soup completely before refrigerating so that it doesn't go sour.

PS. If you cannot have cheese you can substitute it with tofu. It may not be quite as tasty, however, but it will be nutritious.

# SALADS AND SALAD DRESSINGS

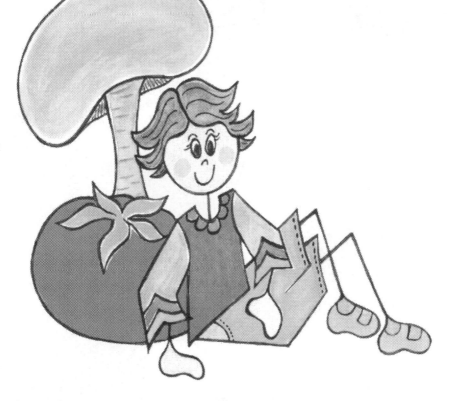

## SPINACH SALAD

1 Lb. of mozzarella cheese or goat cheese
1 Lb. of spinach (see Before You Start Cooking)
2 Lbs. of tomato peeled and seeded
3 Red bell peppers roasted and peeled (see Before You Start Cooking)
4 cloves of garlic, pureed or finely chopped
Extra virgin olive oil or grape seed oil
Salt and ground black pepper to taste

Prepare the spinach as indicated in the tip section. Because this is for a salad remember to place the spinach in icy water to stop the cooking process, keeping it crunchy. Also remember to strain any excess water. Finely chop the spinach, dice the roasted pepper and the tomato and cut the cheese into squares. Mix all the ingredients together. Add the garlic and the olive oil and mix well. Serve cold.


## FRUIT SALAD WITH CORN

2 Cups of cooked green beans (cut in, half inch segments)
2 ½ Cups of Uchuvas (*Physalis Peruviana L.*) sliced in half (in a pinch you can use any berry))
2 Cups tangerine sections (if using fresh remove pips)
1 Lb. of whole corn kernels (cooked) or you can use frozen
1 ½ tbsp. grated and then finely chopped fresh ginger
1 ½ Cups of roughly chopped cashew nuts (or any other nut)
¼ Cup honey
1 Cup sour cream

In a large bowl mix the corn, green beans, Uchuvas , tangerine sections, ½ tsp. of the ginger and half of the honey (1/8 of a cup). Mix the remaining honey and ginger with the sour cream. Add the nuts to the salad just before serving so that they do not loose their crunch. Place a spoonful of the sour cream mixture on top of each serving. Serve cold.


## RED SALAD

6 large beetroots cooked and diced
1½ Cups strawberries
1 Cup blueberries
1 ½ Cups sliced almonds
1 ½ Cups sour cream
1 Cup chopped mint leaves
1 tbsp. honey
1/8 Cup of strawberry vinegar (or cider vinegar)
Salt
Ground black pepper (the more the better)

Marinate the beetroot with vinegar, honey and salt for about a half an hour. Toast the almonds on a tray in the oven till golden in color. Mix half of the chopped mint with the sour cream. Strain the beetroot and mix with the strawberries, the blueberries, the remaining chopped mint and the ground pepper. Serve a spoonful of the sour cream and mint mixture over each serving and garnish with the toasted almonds.


## MANGO SALAD

1 ½ Cups of cooked red pinto beans
3 large mangos (ripe but firm to the touch)
12 radishes
1 bunch of watercress trimmed and coarsely chopped
1 large avocado (firm, not over ripe)

1 Lb. mozzarella cheese or goat cheese
2 Cups chopped cilantro
¼ Cup extra virgin olive oil
1 tbsp. extra virgin olive oil
4 tbsp. lime juice
¼ Cup honey
Salt
1 head of romaine lettuce

Marinate the cooked red beans with 1 tablespoon of lime juice, salt and 1 tablespoon of extra virgin olive oil. Peel and dice the mango. Set aside ½ a cup of mango for the dressing. Peel and slice the avocado. Cut cheese in squares. Cut radishes in half and thinly slice. Mix all these ingredients in a large bowl and refrigerate while you prepare the dressing.

Place the cilantro, the ¼ Cup of extra virgin olive oil, the remaining 3 tbsp. lemon juice, the honey and the ½ Cup of mango that was set aside, in the blender and blend till smooth. Arrange each serving of salad on a piece of lettuce and drizzle with dressing.

## BARLEY SALAD

5 Cups of cooked barley
3 avocados peeled and sliced
1 Cup sliced black olives
2 Cups of sliced mushrooms (washed)
2 cloves of garlic (pureed) or finely chopped
1 Lb goat cheese cut in squares
1 large red onion diced
2 large red bell peppers roasted and chopped (see Before You Start Cooking)
¼ Cup olive oil

Salt
Ground black pepper

Sautee the mushrooms for about 1 minute in a little of the olive oil and a dash of salt and pepper. Add the garlic and cook for a few minutes. In a large bowl mix all the ingredients including the cooled mushrooms. Refrigerate before serving.

## ARRACACHA AND PINEAPPLE SALAD

Arracacha: celery root, or sometimes called white carrot, has a slight celery flavor and a potato consistency.

3 Cups of cooked and cubed Arracacha (It can most likely be found in a latin supermarket)
1 Cup of finely chopped red onion
1 ½ Cups of fresh or canned pineapple (without liquid)
1 ½ Cups of coarsely chopped celery
¼ Cup extra virgin olive oil
1 Tbsp. vinegar
Salt
Freshly ground black pepper

Note: When cooking the Arracacha be careful not to overcook. It cooks in a" blink of an eye".

In a large bowl stir the onion, celery, vinegar, olive oil and the salt and pepper together. Marinate for about ½ an hour. Add the pineapple and the Arracacha to the rest of the ingredients and mix. Serve cold.

# ARRACACHA AND POMELO SALAD

For this salad you must first peel the pomelo (citrus family, about the size of a grapefruit with its own distinctive flavor, sweet and tart). Remove the skin, pips and pith (very thick) and membrane. Cut sections into bite size pieces. Proceed with the same instructions as the previous recipe, replacing the pineapple with the Pomelo. Serve cold.

# TOFU SALAD

2 Cups tofu cut into squares
½ Cup finely chopped onion
2 Cups diced tomatoes, peeled and seeded (see Before You Start Cooking)
1 Cup chopped cilantro
2 Cups romaine lettuce, julienned
3 cloves of garlic pureed (more or less depending on your tastes)
1 tbsp soy sauce
1 tbsp lemon juice (more or less, your choice)
¼ Cup extra virgin olive oil
¼ tsp turmeric powder (optional)
Salt and freshly ground black pepper to taste

Whisk together the olive oil, lemon juice, pureed garlic, turmeric, chopped onion, soy sauce, salt and pepper. Gently toss the tofu with the above mixture and set aside in the refrigerator to marinate, at least 15 minutes or till ready to serve. To serve gently toss the lettuce and the tomato with the tofu mixture. Have this with a corn tortilla or pita bread or just as is. Delish!

## SMOKED SAUCE OR SALSA

2 large red bell peppers roasted (see TIP section)
6 large firm ripe tomatoes
2 whole heads of garlic
3 tbsp. extra virgin olive oil
Salt
Ground black pepper

Place the tomatoes over a flame turning till all sides are charred as when roasting a pepper. Roast the red peppers following the instructions in the Before You Start Cooking section. Place the garlic over a very, very low flame and turn slowly till the garlic feels soft to the touch. Peel and seed the tomatoes and squeeze out all the water. Peel and seed the pimentos and peel the garlic cloves squeezing out the buttery pulp. Process all the ingredients with the olive oil the salt and the ground black pepper. Serve as a salsa for tortillas or chips, for seasoning your tofu and gluten or just spreading it on your sandwiches.

## TARTAR SAUCE (" VEGGIE" VERSION )

1 ½ Cups of sour cream
1 Cup parsley, thoroughly washed and finely chopped
2 cucumbers peeled, seeded and finely chopped
1 Cup of finely chopped spring onion
3 cloves of garlic pureed
Salt
Ground black pepper

Place the peeled, seeded and very finely chopped cucumber in a sieve and set aside for a couple of hours. This is to drain all the water from the cucumber.  Now add the cucumber, chopped parsley, onion, garlic, salt and pepper to the sour cream and stir thoroughly. Keep refrigerated till ready to use.

P.S.  This was my Mom's way of making tartar sauce.  Of course she used mayonnaise.  If you prefer, you can make your own mayonnaise without egg, but I think that the sour cream does the trick and saves time.  Either way, go for it.

Good, just as a salad dressing, a dip or as a sauce for sandwiches and veggie burgers. Very light and refreshing.

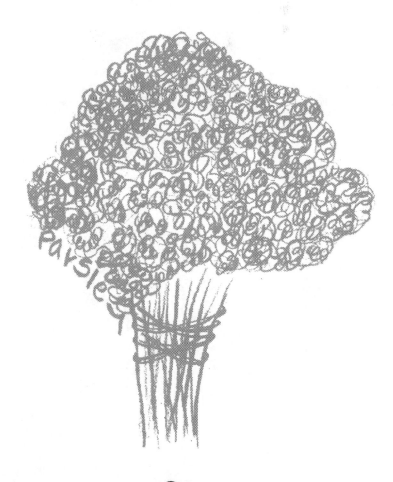

# FUN FOOD (BUT HEALTHY)

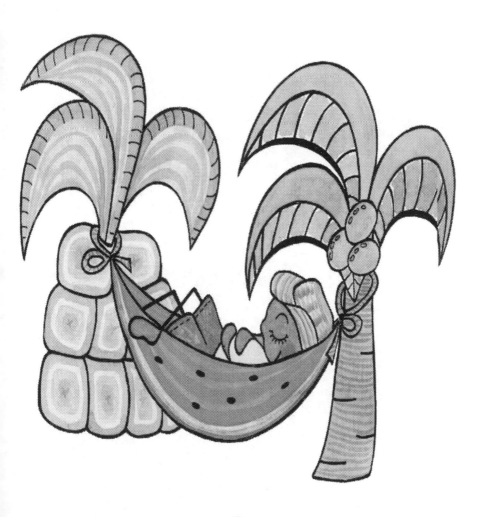

# EGGLESS CARROT SOUFFLÉ

4 Carrots cooked and grated (2 cups)
2 Tbsp. capers
1 large onion finely diced (1 cup)
8 slices of old whole wheat bread (2 cups
1 Lb. Spanish style white cheese or goat cheese
1 Cup of milk
Salt
Freshly ground black pepper
Extra virgin olive oil or grape seed oil

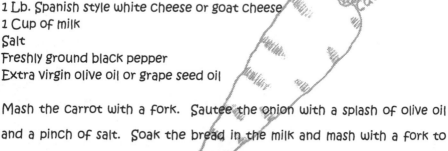

Mash the carrot with a fork. Sautee the onion with a splash of olive oil and a pinch of salt. Soak the bread in the milk and mash with a fork to break up the bread. Grate the cheese and mix all the ingredients together. Pour the soufflé into a greased baking dish and bake in 200°C (400°F) oven for 30 minutes or till cooked and golden in color

P.S. It is better if you mix everything with your hands. Messy but better.

# SLOPPY JOES

2 Cups TVP (see TIP section)
1 ½ Lb. tomato peeled, seeded and finely chopped or processed
5 cloves of garlic, mashed
2 medium carrots peeled and grated
1 tsp sugar
½ head of lettuce shredded
1 Cup Gouda cheese, grated  (any strong flavored yellow cheese will do)
2 tbsp cornstarch
Salt
Ground black pepper
Extra virgin olive oil
6 hamburger buns

Prepare the TVP as indicated in the Before You Start Cooking section. Mix the tomato, the carrot, the garlic, the TVP, the sugar, a splash of olive oil, salt and pepper in a saucepot and simmer till most of the liquid has evaporated. Dissolve the cornstarch in a little bit of water. Remove the pot from the burner, stir in the dissolved cornstarch, return the pot to the burner and simmer till the cornstarch is cooked and the sauce has thickened.

Serve a spoonful on each bun and add the cheese and the lettuce on top.

## ONION AND LEEK PIE

4 white or yellow onions
5 leeks
½ Cup grated Gouda or Cheddar cheese
4 tbsp extra virgin olive oil
1 tbsp flour
3 tbsp sour cream
1 Cup parmesan cheese
3 Cup fresh bread crumbs
Salt
Ground black pepper
2 Tbsp butter
Pie pastry (see "Dessert Basics ")

Cut onions in half and slice. Fry till golden. Cut the white part of the leeks in slices (wash very well) and sauté till tender. Mix both onions together with the flour, the grated Gouda, the salt and pepper and the sour cream.

Make pastry. Roll out the dough with a rolling pin and make a circle to fit a nine inch pie pan. Fill the pastry with the onion filling. Mix the breadcrumbs, the parmesan and the butter together with your fingers to achieve a uniform crumble. Sprinkle over the top of the onion filling, pressing down lightly with your hand. Bake in a 200°C (400°F) oven for about 40 minutes. Remember to preheat your oven (see Dessert Basics).


## "NO-FISH-CAKES"

This is a teeny tiny recipe so just double up on the ingredients when you need to feed a larger crowd.

1 Cup oatmeal (flakes)
2 Tbsp grated onion
1 cloves of garlic mashed
1 1/2 Cups Milk
2 Tbsp Flour
1 Tsp thyme
1 Tsp sage
Salt and ground black pepper
Grape seed oil or extra virgin olive oil for frying
Extra flour for flouring the patties

Mix one cup of milk, the sage, the thyme, the salt and pepper with the flour and place in a small sauce pot over medium heat. Bring to the boil stirring constantly. Remove from heat when mixture bubbles and thickens. Add the oatmeal, the garlic and the onion. Stir thoroughly. This will make about 8, ¼ inch patties or you can of course make the patties larger but you should always make them ¼ of an inch thick so that they cook through. Place each patty in the remaining ½ cup of milk and then in the flour, coating on all sides. Fry in a non stick frying pan with a little oil till golden and crispy.

## SWEET POTATO PUREE

1 Lb. sweet potato cooked
1 Lb. ñame (also known as Oca or *Oxalis tuberose* — tubers). You can probably buy it in a latin supermarket, or you can substitute with potato
2 Cups of plain yogurt
½ tsp salt
1 ½ Cups sliced or slivered almonds toasted
¼ Cup of raw or brown sugar
3 tbsp of butter

Peel, cook and mash the ñame (or potato) and the sweet potato. You can use a fork or potato masher to mash the ñame and the sweet potato. Add the salt, yogurt, sugar and butter mixing well. Sprinkle the toasted almonds over each serving or place in a serving dish and sprinkle the toasted almonds over top.

P.S A personal tip: A potato peeler will peel the thick ñame skin easily

Be careful, peeled ñame is slippery.

## BAKED EMPANADAS

An empanada is a half moon shaped pastry, to be eaten with your hands.

Dough recipe for all of the following empanadas

4 Cups all purpose flour
1 Cup milk

¾ Cup butter
¼ tsp salt
2 tsp mixed herbs (oregano, thyme, rosemary, Italian blend, French blend, etc.)

Heat the milk, butter and salt and add to the flour. Knead with your hands and divide in 10 equal balls of dough. ( For bigger empanadas divide dough into 6 or 8 balls) With a rolling pin, roll out each ball of dough, on a floured surface, into a 1/8 of an inch thick circle. Fill one half of the circle with one tenth of the filling. Wet the edges with a little milk and fold the opposite side of the circle over the filling and press down the edges with a fork. Cut excess dough with a knife. Bake on a greased tray in a 200°C (400°F) oven for about 45 minutes.

## SWISS CHARD EMPANADA FILLING:

2 Lb. Swiss chard cooked and chopped and
1 Cup finely chopped white or yellow onion
¾ Lb. mozzarella or Spanish style white cheese (grated)
½ Cup parmesan
3 tbsp flour
Extra virgin olive oil
Salt and ground black pepper

Drain as much of the water from the cooked chard as you can. Sautee the onion with a little olive oil and add to the chard together with the flour stirring well. Fold in the cheese. Prepare and bake as indicated previously in the **BAKED EMPANADAS** recipe.

## CHILEAN EMPANADA FILLING:

3 tbsp small capers
3 Cups sliced onions
½ Cup raisins

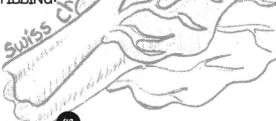

16 whole kalamata olives or ½ CUP sliced olives of choice
1 Lb. gluten diced or 3 Cups of hydrated TVP (see Before You Start Cooking)
2 tbsp soy sauce
1 tbsp caper brine
½ tsp turmeric powder
2 tsp curry powder, optional
2 tbsp flour
Extra virgin olive oil
Salt and fresh ground black pepper

Toss the diced gluten or the TVP with the flour and stir fry in olive oil to brown. Fry the onions until golden in color. Mix the gluten or TVP, raisins, olives, onions, soy sauce, turmeric, capers, caper brine, curry powder, salt and pepper. Note: These empanadas can be seasoned with the curry but are also tasty without. This is why the curry powder is included as optional. Both ways are good. Prepare and bake as indicated in the **BAKED EMPANADAS** recipe.

## GLUTEN PITA POCKETS

½ a medium size head of lettuce
6 tomatoes diced (see Before You Start Cooking)
3 tbsp soy sauce
3 cloves of garlic mashed
1 Lb. gluten julienned
Tarter sauce (see Salads and Salad Dressings)
Corn flour
4 pita breads cut in half
½ Lb. of firm Spanish style white cheese

Rinse and shred the lettuce and set aside. Season the gluten with the soy sauce and the garlic and marinate for ½ an hour. Place the corn flour in a bag, add the seasoned gluten and toss till coated. Place on greased tray and bake for 20 minutes till crispy. Set aside. Grate the cheese and set aside. Cut the pita breads in half to make the pockets. Add a little of the tarter sauce in the bottom of each pocket, some of the lettuce, some gluten, some tomato, a little more tarter sauce and the cheese. This will be enough for 4 or 8 people depending on their appetites.


## PLANTAIN BAKE

4 ripe plantains diced
1 Lb. Spanish style white cheese grated
2 tbsp brown or raw sugar (optional)
1 tsp cinnamon
1/3 cup + 1 tbsp milk
4 tbsp flour
¼ tsp baking soda
Extra virgin olive oil or grape seed oil

Fry the diced plantain in a non stick pan with a little oil till golden. Add the sugar, cinnamon, flour, baking soda, the milk and the cheese. Fold in the ingredients. Bake in greased baking dish in a 200°C (400°F) oven for 25 minutes.


## KEDGEREE

1 Lb. cherry tomatoes cut in half
3 cups of hydrated TVP (see Before You Start Cooking))
1 cup raisins
1 cup capers
½ cup green olives sliced
1 cup whole black olives

4 red onions diced
1/4 cup soy sauce
2 tsp balsamic vinegar
1 tsp tomato paste
Ground black pepper
Extra virgin olive oil

Fry the onions in a little olive oil till caramelized. Add raisins, black pepper, capers, green and black olives and the TVP, stirring well. Toss the tomatoes with the balsamic vinegar, tomato paste and a little olive oil. Add to previous mixture stirring well and heating thoroughly. Serve with rice.


## GRILLED PINEAPPLE PITAS

4 pita breads cut in half
2 tbsp honey
2 tbsp melted butter
4 slices of fresh pineapple cut in half
4 Thick slices of mozzarella

Light the grill, gas or charcoal. Mix the honey with the butter, paint one side of each slice of pineapple and place on the grill. Turn over and paint with butter and honey mixture. Remove from the Grill when caramelized and with the crisscrossed grill marks. Place a slice of cheese on each piece of hot pineapple so that the cheese can melt. Cut each cheese-and-pineapple-combo in half and slide each half into half a pita pocket. Warm the pineapple pitas on the grill for a few seconds before serving. Enjoy.

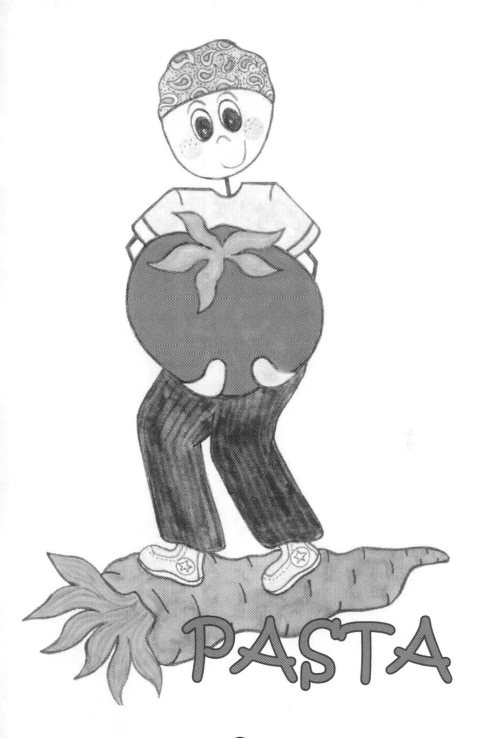

PASTA

# ROASTED RED PEPPER PASTA

1 Lb. pasta of your choice
4 large red bell peppers roasted (see Before You Start Cooking)
4 large tomatoes peeled and seeded (see Before You Star Cooking)
2 large red onions diced
1 Lb. sliced mushrooms
5 cloves of garlic pureed or finely chopped
2 bay leaves
2 tbsp chopped fresh oregano
Salt and ground black pepper to taste.
Extra virgin olive oil
Grated Romano cheese

Prepare the peppers. Process or blend the roasted peppers and the tomatoes. Fry the onions for 2 minutes in a little olive oil then add the pureed garlic, salt pepper and the mushrooms and sauté for 2 minutes. Add the blended pimento and tomato. Add the bay leaf and the oregano and simmer on low heat for 5 minutes. Serve over the cooked pasta sprinkled with some grated Romano cheese. Remove the bay leaf.

# ROSEMARY PASTA

1 Lb. Pasta of your choice
3 tbsp of chopped fresh rosemary
1 Cup cream
1 Cup parmesan grated parmesan cheese
1 Lb. tomatoes diced (see Before You Start Cooking))

1 Cup diced white or yellow onion
3 Cups finely chopped spinach (see Before You Start Cooking))
¼ Cup extra virgin olive oil
Salt and ground black pepper

Sauté the onion with olive oil for 2 minutes, add the tomato and sauté for 2 more minutes. Add the spinach and simmer for 2 more minutes.

Fold the parmesan and the rosemary into the cream

Cook the pasta according to directions. Spoon sauce over pasta and add a dollop of the sour cream mixture over top.

## WHITE WINE PASTA

1 Lb. pasta
2 white or Spanish onions diced
½ Lb. sliced mushrooms
1 Cup smoked Tilsit or Gouda cheese grated (or any other smoked cheese)
1 Cup parmesan grated
1 Cup mozzarella cut into small cubes
4 Cups milk
5 tbsp corn starch
2 Cups of white wine
1 tsp sugar
Ground black pepper
Salt
Extra virgin olive oil

Sauté the onions 1 minute then add the mushrooms and sauté for 2 more minutes. Stir in the salt, the sugar, the pepper and the wine and simmer 2 more minutes. Dissolve the corn starch first in a little milk and add to the mushroom mixture with the rest of the milk stirring over medium heat till mixture thickens. Fold in the cheese, the parmesan and the mozzarella.

Serve hot over the pasta of choice.

## THAI PASTA

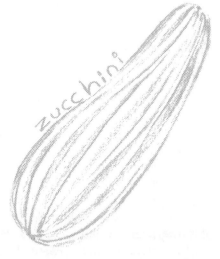

1 Lb. rice noodles
1 Lb. carrots julienne or matchstick
1 Lb. zucchini julienne or matchstick
2 Cups spring onion cut in 1 inch pieces
2 Cups orange juice
2 tbsp ginger grated and finely chopped
3 tbsp soy sauce
½ Cup Peanut butter
1 tbsp honey
¾ Cup sesame seeds toasted
Sesame seed oil

Toast the sesame in a nonstick frying pan on low heat for 3 minutes stirring constantly and set aside. Whisk the orange juice, soy sauce and the peanut butter and the grated ginger till blended. Stir fry the carrots, in the sesame oil, till crunchy and tender. Stir fry the zucchini the same way. Mix the carrots, zucchini and the spring onion and stir fry together for another minute. Add the peanut butter sauce and heat thoroughly.

Serve over rice noodles and sprinkle with toasted sesame seeds.

## "WACHAMACALLIT" PASTA

1 Lb. noodles
1 Lb. Spanish Style white cheese diced
¼ Lb. Gouda Cheese, grated
3 Lbs. tomato prepared for sauce peeled, seeded, strained and diced. (see Before You Start Cooking )

1 Cup pitted olives
1 Cup coarsely chopped fresh basil
Extra virgin olive oil
Salt and ground black pepper

Mix the tomato, olives, the diced white cheese, the shredded Gouda, basil, olive oil and the salt and pepper all together. Cook and strain pasta. Mix all the raw ingredients while the pasta is piping hot. Serve immediately.

## PASTA FOR EGGPLANT LOVERS

1 Lb. pasta of choice
5 cloves of garlic pureed or finely chopped
2 Lbs. eggplant peeled and diced (see Before You Start Cooking)
2 Lbs. tomato diced (see Before You Start Cooking)
1 ½ Cup sliced black olives
½ Cup finely chopped fresh basil
4 tbsp extra virgin olive oil
Salt
Fresh ground pepper
Parmesan or Romano cheese

Dice and toss the prepared eggplant with half the olive oil and ¼ Cup water and bake on a cookie sheet in a 200°C (400 °F) oven till tender. Cook pasta according to package instructions and strain. Pour the remaining half of the olive oil in a saucepan and sauté the tomato and the garlic for 3 to 4 minutes. Now mix all the ingredients and simmer for a couple more minutes. Serve the eggplant sauce over the hot pasta. Add cheese to each serving.

# HEART WARMING DISHES

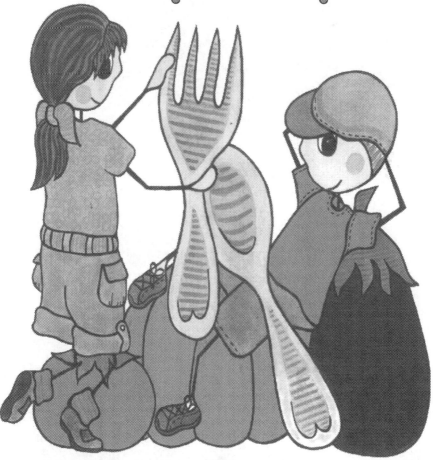

# CURRIED POTATOES MY WAY

2 white or yellow onions
8 Celery stalks
1 Cup plain unsweetened yogurt
1 tsp raw or brown sugar
6 large potatoes
Extra virgin olive oil
1 tsp curry powder (more or less depending on how hot you like it)
Salt
Freshly ground green pepper corns

Cut the celery into bite size pieces and slice the onion. Stir fry together for 3 minutes with the curry powder. Add the yogurt, the sugar, the onion, the salt and the ground green pepper to the celery and curry mixture. Cut the potatoes into bite size pieces, and boil in salted water till they are par (A little raw) cooked. Drain the water and mix with the curried vegetable mixture. Cook for a couple of minutes till potatoes are cooked. Serve hot. Note: Leaving the potatoes slightly under cooked is to prevent them from breaking up when cooking with the vegetables.

# STROGANOFF

1 Lb. of gluten or Tofu
1 Lb. of fresh mushrooms sliced
2 tbsp sherry or brandy
1 Cup parsley washed and finely chopped
2 Cups of white or yellow onion fine diced
2 tbsp soy sauce
1 clove garlic pureed
½ tsp Dijon mustard
1 Cup corn flour
Extra virgin olive oil
Salt and ground black pepper

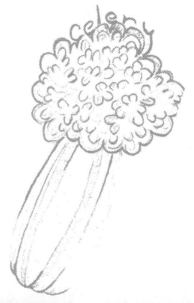

Cut the gluten in cubes and season with soy sauce, 1 tbsp olive oil and garlic. Place corn flour in plastic bag, add the gluten and toss till it is evenly coated. Discard excess corn flour. Spread evenly on a greased tray and bake in a 200°C (400°F) oven till golden but not dried out (about 15 minutes). Sauté the onion in a little olive oil for one minute then add the mushrooms and sauté for 2 minutes more. Add the gluten, the mustard, the cream, and the parsley and simmer for 2 minutes. Last but not least add the sherry and stir thoroughly. Note: When boiled, spirits lose their alcohol content leaving just the flavor. Serve hot with rice or noodles.

## CORN BAKE

8 Cups whole fresh corn kernels (or frozen)
1 Cup cream
1 ½ cups firm white Spanish style cheese grated
2 Lbs. tomato coarsely chopped (see Before You Start Cooking)
4 Cups peas (frozen or canned)
1 Lb. gluten
4 tbsp corn flour
1/8 Cup sugar
¼ Cup melted butter
Extra virgin olive oil
Salt and freshly ground black pepper

Grease an oven proof dish and set aside. Cut the gluten into small bite size pieces and season with the soy sauce, garlic, olive oil and pepper. Marinate for 10 to 15 minutes. Place in a bag with the corn flour and toss till coated. Remove excess corn flour and place on a greased cookie sheet and bake for 15 minutes or till golden. Put the corn in the processor and pulse till pureed. Add the grated cheese, the cream and the butter. Pulse till blended.. Set aside. Sauté the onion with a little olive oil for 2 minutes then add the tomato, the gluten and the peas. Simmer for 3 to 4 minutes more. Cover the bottom of a greased baking dish with half of the corn mixture. Spread the tomato and gluten mixture evenly over this. Now top with the remaining corn mixture.

Bake at a 175°C (350 °F) for 45 min. to an hour.

## STUFFED MUSHROOMS

4 large Portobello mushrooms
1 Cup parmesan or pecorino cheese grated
6 Cups fresh bread crumbs
¼ Cup chopped parsley
1 white or yellow onion finely chopped
1 Tbsp. sherry
2 Tbsp. heavy cream
Extra virgin olive oil
Salt
Freshly ground black pepper

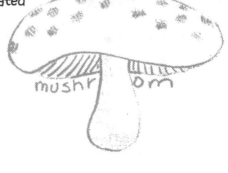

Wash and dry the mushrooms. Remove the stalks and chop finely. Sautee the finely chopped Portobello stalks and the chopped onion for a couple of minutes. Add the parsley, the bread crumbs, the sherry, the cream, the cheese, the salt and the freshly ground black pepper and thoroughly mix. Divide the mixture in four and fill each mushroom. Place the mushrooms in a baking dish with about ½ a cup of water, a pinch of salt and 1 tbsp olive oil. Bake at 200°C (400°F), for half an hour or till the mushrooms are cooked and the cheese is a nice golden color.

PS: You can make fresh bread crumbs by placing slices of bread in a processor or blender.

## SWEET AND SOUR VEGGIES WITH TOFU

1 Lb. tofu cut into bite size pieces
2 medium zucchini cut in half and sliced
1 small broccoli cut into bite size pieces
1 large green bell pepper cut into slivers (not too thin)
2 celery stalks cut into bite size pieces (not too thin)
1 medium carrot cut into slivers (not too thin)
3 Cups pineapple grilled and cut into bite size pieces
3 tbsp pineapple juice
½ Lb. package of baby corn
1 Tbsp grated fresh ginger
2 Tbsp lemon juice
½ grated lemon peel
1 ½ tbsp honey
1 ½ Cups cashew nuts, chopped
3 Tbsp. corn starch
¼ Cup soy sauce
Salt
Freshly ground black pepper
Toasted sesame oil

Stir fry each of the following ingredients, individually, in the toasted sesame oil; Zucchini for 1 minute, broccoli 3 minutes, celery 2 minutes and carrots 2 minutes. Deep fat fry the tofu till crispy. Drain well on paper towels. In a large pot stir the honey, soy sauce, grated ginger and lemon juice, freshly ground black pepper to taste and the grated lemon peel. Now add all the vegetables and tofu and stir. Mix the corn starch with the pineapple juice. Mix in with the vegetables and cook till liquid thickens.  Serve hot over rice or with noodles and sprinkle with the chopped nuts.


## WHOLE-GRAIN RICE CASSEROLE

2 Cups whole-grain rice (un-cooked)
1 Tbsp. soy sauce
¼ Cup grape seed oil or canola oil
1/ Lb. grated parmesan cheese
1 ½ Cup black olives without pips and sliced
4 Medium size zucchinis cut in half and sliced
8 fresh artichoke hearts (see Before You Start Cooking) or use canned
2 ½ Lbs. tomatoes (see Before You Start Cooking)) diced
2 eggplants (see Before You Start Cooking)) diced
3 Cups mozzarella diced or any similar cheese diced
1 tsp sugar
Salt and freshly ground black pepper

Add rice, salt and oil to a heavy saucepot and stir fry on low to medium heat till rice toasts to a nice golden color.  Be careful not to burn.  This may take about 5 minutes.  Add 6 cups of water and the soy sauce and boil slowly till most of the water evaporates, not completely. Now cover and lower the heat, very low and leave untouched for about 20 minutes.  Now with a large spoon turn the rice over evenly and cover the pot once again and cook for another 10 minutes.  When the rice has cooled completely put it in the processor and pulse till the rice is coarsely  ground .  Add the parmesan cheese mixing well. Line a baking pan with the cheese and rice mixture and bake in a 200°C (400 °F) oven for half an hour or till it gets a nice golden color.

Stir fry the zucchini in hot skillet for about a minute and set aside in colander to strain. Stir fry the eggplant in the skillet till cooked. Cut the artchokes into bite size pieces. Mix the olives and all the vegetables and simmer for 1 minute. Add the sugar, the salt and pepper to taste and the mozzarella cheese. Spoon this mixture evenly over the previously baked rice mixture. Place in a 200°C (400°F) for 40 minutes.

## TVP CHILE (Tastes better than it sounds, honest.)

4 red onions diced
2 Lbs. tomato (see Tip section) coarsely chopped
2 Cups whole corn kernels
2 Cups hydrated TVP (textured vegetable protein)
4 cloves of garlic
2 Tbsp. chili powder (more or less)
1 ½ raw or brown sugar
2 Tbsp soy sauce
4 Cups cooked red beans, reserve 1 cup of the water used to cook the beans
Salt
Grape seed or canola oil

Fry the onion in a little oil till cooked. Add the garlic, sugar, chili powder, corn and tomato and simmer for 3 minutes. Add the TVP and simmer 3 minutes more. Add the beans, the bean water, soy sauce and salt if necessary. Simmer 4 minutes or more, uncovered, till some of the liquid evaporates and mixture thickens. Yummy with whole grain rice!

# ETOUFFE

1 Lb. of mushrooms cut up into chunky pieces
3 Tbsp. butter
5 cloves of garlic pureed
3 celery stalks with leaves, coarsely chopped
3 Tbsp. flour
1 ½ Cups chopped spring onion
1 ½ Cups of finely chopped parsley
1 white or yellow onion finely diced
2 ½ Cups milk
1½ Cups water
Freshly ground black pepper
Hot pepper flakes optional
Salt

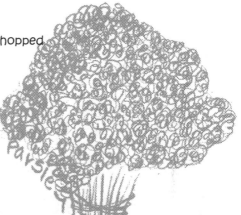

I was told this is a Cajun dish but for vegetarian purposes I have modified it. We all enjoy it this way very much.

Heat butter in frying pan, add the chopped white onion and sauté for 1 minute. Add the mushrooms and stir fry for another 2 minutes. Add the garlic and salt to taste. Stir fry for 1 minute longer. Put the chopped celery and the water in a pot and simmer, with the lid on, for 5 minutes on medium heat. Blend the cooked celery and the water in a blender and strain. Put the strained celery liquid and milk back in the blender with the flour and blend once more. Put the liquid in a pot and cook till mixture is creamy. Mix the sautéed onion and mushroom mixture, the chopped spring onion and the finely chopped parsley with the creamy celery soup. Add the black pepper or the hot pepper flakes. Stir well and heat thoroughly on low heat. Stir frequently so that the mixture does not stick to the bottom of the pot and burn. Serve over a bowl of hot whole grain rice.

# YUCCA BAKE

2 Lb. yucca
8 tomatoes finely chopped (see Before You Start Cooking)
2 Cups crumbled hard tofu or 2 Cups hydrated TVP (see Before You Start Cooking)
1 Lb. frozen corn kernels
3 white onions diced
5 cloves of garlic pureed
¼ Cup extra virgin olive oil
2 Tbsp. butter
¾ Cup milk
10 black olives
½ Cup chopped cilantro
2 Cups parmesan or pecorino cheese

Stir fry the onion in a little olive oil till golden in color. Add the tomato and the garlic and sauté for 2 minutes. Now add the tofu or TVP, corn, black olives, cilantro and salt and pepper to taste stirring well. Peel and cut the yucca and boil in a large pot with plenty of water and some salt. When done mash the yucca coarsely with a fork and add the milk and butter. Put half of this mixture in the bottom of a baking dish spreading evenly. Pour the tomato mixture in and cover with the remaining pureed yucca. Top with the grated cheese. Bake in a 200°C (400°F) oven for 30 to 40 minutes.

# VEGGIE CASSEROLE

For this recipe feel free to substitute milk for veggie **stock.**

5 medium potatoes sliced
10 pearl onions or any other small onion
1 large carrot cut down the middle length wise and sliced
1 medium zucchini cut down the middle length wise and sliced
1 Cup frozen corn
1 Cup frozen peas
2 Cups diced Spanish style white cheese
1 ½ Cups grated parmesan cheese
½ Cup all purpose flour
2 Cups milk
3 Cups vegetable stock (If you prefer, eliminate the 2 cups of milk and use instead, a total of 5 cups of vegetable stock)
2 tsp dried dill
Salt and freshly ground black pepper

Fill a medium size pot with 3 cups of vegetable stock and add the potatoes and the onions. Boil till potatoes are slightly undercooked. Take out the potatoes and the onions. Now add the carrot, the peas, and the corn. Cover and boil for three minutes. Add the zucchini and cook for one minute. In a small bowl mix the flour with some of the milk. Now mix the milk and flour mixture, the rest of the milk, the pepper and the dill with the vegetables and vegetable stock (not the potato and the onion) and bring to a slow boil till mixture is creamy. At this point add the parmesan, stirring well. Cover the bottom of a large baking dish with the potatoes, the diced white cheese and the onions and cover with the creamed vegetable mixture. Bake in a 175°C or (350°F) oven for about ½ an hour. Broil for a few minutes to brown the top a little.

# CURRIED POTATOES A LA MAHARAJAH

This recipe was inspired by a very dear friend. Thank you. We always enjoy it very much.

5 potatoes cut into small bite sized pieces
3 large tomatoes, peeled, seeded and finely diced
2 medium onions thinly sliced
2 cloves of garlic (mashed)
¼ Cup olive oil
1 Tbsp. curry powder (add more or less according to taste. 1 Tbsp is spicy)

1 Tbsp. dark soy sauce
Salt

Add oil to a medium size heavy pot. Heat over medium heat and add the onion. Sauté for ½ a minute, then add the garlic and the tomato and sauté for 1 more minute. Add the potato and the soy sauce and continue sautéing over medium to low heat stirring constantly for 2 or three minutes. Cover and simmer over low heat, stirring often till the potatoes are cooked but juicy. If the mixture looks like it is drying out or sticking too much, add a little bit of water. Serve this with a tomato, lettuce and pineapple salad. The combination of the curried potatoes and the pineapple in the salad is refreshing.

Tomato

# DESSERT BASICS

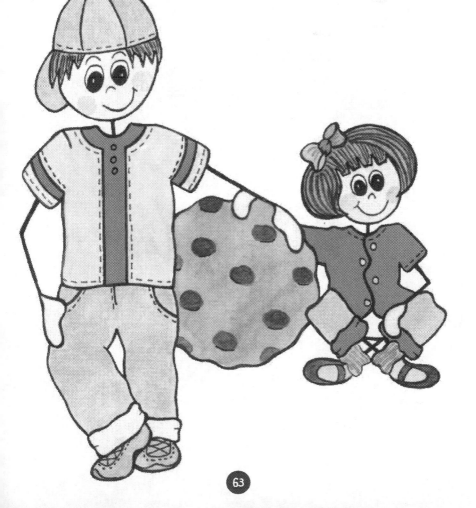

## GOOD RECOMMENDATIONS FOR MAKING CAKES

1. On a personal note, I like to use a cheesecake pan or pan with a removable bottom for making cakes. This makes it easier to get the cake out. You can also use a Teflon liner or wax paper, cut to the size of the pan. Any of these solutions will work.

2. When filling your cake pan make sure not to fill to the top. Fill to about ¾ of the pan. This goes for muffins or cupcakes too.

## NO EGGS IN THIS COOKBOOK

I have nothing against eggs, you guys, but I just do not use them.

On this note I just wanted to repeat what I have already mentioned in the "Before You Start Cooking Section". I substitute ¼ Cup Yogurt for each egg that is scratched from a recipe. You can also use 1 Tbsp of vinegar for one egg you eliminate or 2 tablespoons for 2 eggs you eliminate. A recipe that calls for 3 eggs or more is best not messing with.

## MEASURING CUPS

Use the same set of measuring cups. Not to long ago I was making pastry and I had two different sets of measuring cups. Thinking they were "all created equal", I used both sets for the same recipe. The mixture did not come out right and I could not figure out why. It occurred to me to check to see if the cups measured the same and to my surprise they did not. So now I am careful to only use one set at a time.

## FOLLOW THESE STEPS WHEN BAKING

a. Preheat oven 15 to 20 minutes before baking

b. Cooking time can depend on geographic location. Sea level or otherwise. For instance, I live on the Colombian coast and my baking time is totally different to baking time in Bogota which is 3000 meters higher.

c. Use a toothpick, metal skewer or, as I recently learned, a piece of thin uncooked pasta to test if the cakes are done. When the toothpick comes out clean or when the cake pulls away from the sides of the pan the cake is done.

d. As mentioned before do not overfill the cake pan. Fill ¾ of the way up.

e. Let cake cool for about 10 minutes before removing from pan.

f. When cutting layers in half, horizontally, make sure the cake has completely cooled. If you have the time, freeze the cake. This makes it less likely to break when handling.

g. Different locations, altitudes and ovens make it impossible to determine exact temperatures and cooking time. So..... keep your eye on the baked goods while they are in the oven.

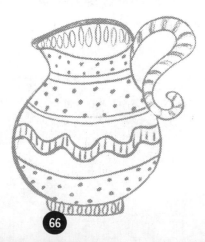

## PIE PASTRY RECIPE

2 Cups of flour
½ Tsp salt
1 Tbsp. sugar
2/3 Cup cold butter
6 to 7 Tbsp. cold water
½ tsp baking powder

In a large bowl mix the flour, salt, baking powder, sugar and the butter cut up in small pieces. You can use your fingers to blend the butter evenly into the flour mixture but it is actually better to use a pastry cutter. Why you may ask? The heat from your fingers melts the butter and the butter should remain as cold as possible. Add the water little by little while tossing the flour mixture with a fork or with the pastry cutter. Depending on the moisture level of the butter you may not need all the allotted water. Your pastry should be firm and moist but not sticky. Too much water makes the pastry tough. You can also make the pastry in the processor if you have one. Put the flour, sugar, salt and sugar and pulse to mix. Now add the cut up butter and pulse once more to mix. Add the water sprinkling it evenly over the flour and butter mixture and pulse several times. This recipe is enough for a 9 inch pie top and bottom or just the bottom of a larger pie plate. Allow the pastry to sit in the refrigerator for a half an hour or more. Divide the dough in two, one portion bigger that the other. Roll the larger ball out with a rolling pin on a floured surface. Eyeball the size for your pie dish. Roll the dough onto the rolling pin to piggyback it to the dish. You can use your fingers but the rolling pin makes it easier. If it tears don't worry about it, it happens. Just patch it up with another piece of pastry. It's at the bottom; nobody is going to see. Practice makes perfect. When you have filled your pie do the same for the top. Cut the excess around the edges and pinch together of press down with a floured fork. Make little slits around the top of the pie to let the steam out. If you feel creative cut shapes out of the remaining dough and decorate. Some pies do not have a pastry top but a crumble topping instead. Next recipe!

# SWEET CRUMBLE TOPPING

1 Cup flour
¾ Cup brown sugar
¼ Cup butter

Mix the flour and the sugar and cut the butter in little pieces, blending the ingredients evenly till it resembles coarse crumbs. Spread this mixture evenly over the pie filling and bake in a 200°C (400°F) oven for 40 minutes or till pastry is golden and flaky .

# SAVORY CRUMBLE TOPPING

1 cup fresh bread crumbs

1 Cup parmesan cheese

3 Tbsp butter

Follow previous recipe (Sweet Crumble Topping) instructions.

You can also make a graham cracker crust for some pies so here is the recipe.

# GRAHAM CRACKER CRUST

1/3 Cup melted butter
1 Tbsp Brown sugar (optional)
1 ¼ Cups graham cracker crumbs

Mix the butter with the sugar and the graham cracker crumbs with a fork or your fingers or just place everything in the processor and pulse to blend.

Spread the mixture over the bottom of the pie plate and press down evenly on the bottom and up the sides. If you are using a larger pie plate halve or double the recipe accordingly. This is enough for a 9 inch pie dish. Bake in 180°C (360°F) for 4 to 5 minutes.

## CHOCOLATE COOKIE CRUST

Repeat the above recipe omitting the sugar and removing, if any, the cream between the cookies.

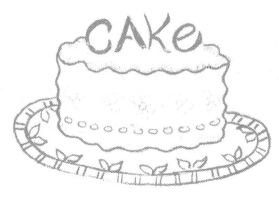

## BASIC VANILLA CAKE

1 1/3 Cups flour
2/3 Cup raw sugar
2 Tsp. baking powder
¼ Tsp. baking soda
2/3 Cup milk
¼ Cup butter (softened)
1 Tsp vanilla
¼ Cup plain yogurt or 1 Tbsp vinegar
¼ Tsp. salt

Mix ( with a whisk) the flour, the sugar, the baking powder, the baking soda and the salt in a bowl. Stir the milk, softened butter, vanilla and yogurt (or vinegar) together and add to the dry ingredients. Whisk or beat at low speed for about 30 seconds. Do not over beat. Grease and flour an 8 x 1 ½ inch pan and bake in 180°C (350°F) oven for 25 minutes or till toothpick comes out clean. Baking time can vary so check on the cake frequently.

When the cake pulls away from the sides of the pan is also an indicator of the cake being done.

## WHIPPED CREAM

2 Cups whipping cream (cold)
1 Tbsp. (or less) sugar
1 large bowl
1 small bowl
Ice

Place small bowl in larger bowl filled with ice and water. Add cream and sugar to small bowl and beat with an electric mixer at high speed or by hand with a whisk (this way can be a little tiring) till peaks form. Be careful not to overbeat because the cream can turn into butter. Keep refrigerated. In a cold climate there is no need for the icy treatment.

## MUFFINS -THE BASIC RECIPE (See more muffin ideas in "DESSERTS"

1 ¾ Cups of flour
1/3 Cup raw sugar or brown sugar
2 Tsp. baking powder
¼ Tsp. baking soda
¾ Cup milk
¼ Cup plain yoghurt
¼ Grape seed or extra virgin olive oil
¼ Tsp. salt
Vanilla or any other essence you choose (for sweet muffins only)

Combine the flour, sugar, baking powder and salt in a bowl and stir with a whisk till thoroughly mixed. In another bowl mix the yoghurt, milk and oil and essence of choice. Add all at once to flour mixture stirring just till moistened. Batter will look lumpy. Grease and flour the muffin pans. Remember as when making cakes only fill 2/3 full. Bake in a 200°C (400°F) oven for 20 minutes. Remove from pans.

You can also add to the recipes as follows:

Idea #1 Apple: dice a cupful and toss with a tsp of flour and a tsp of cinnamon.

Idea #2 Add ½ Cup raisins, or dried cranberries, or chopped prunes, or chopped dates and or ½ Cup chopped nuts

Idea #3. If you want to make a granola muffin add 1 Cup prepared granola or make your own mixture: ¼ Cup rolled oats, ¼ CUP bran and ¼ CUP wheat germ. You can also add ¼ Cup chopped nuts.

Idea #4 Add 1 Cup finely grated carrot and 1 tsp cinnamon.

Idea #5 if you want a cheese muffin you can add 1 Cup grated cheese.

## MUFFIN CUP TIPS

If all the muffin cups are not filled with batter add a little water in each empty space.

## COOKIE TIPS

Cookies are temperamental. You must always keep an eye on them. Do not walk away and ignore them, (who likes to be ignored) if you do, they will probably burn. There is really no way of saying exactly how long they will take, OK. The longer you leave them in (without burning of course) the crunchier they will be. Bake them a little less time and they will be chewy.

I usually always grease my cookie sheet just to be safe. A Teflon or silicon liner, if you have one, is also a good idea.

Wait about a half a minute before removing the cookie from the cookie sheet to let them set up a bit. Do not leave them too long because they may stick to the cookie sheet.

Place cookies on a wire rack to cool.

Cookies baked without eggs tend to get soggy quicker, so place them in an air tight container "ASAP" (as soon as possible).

TRY TO ALWAYS HAVE FUN WHEN COOKING – NEVER LET IT BECOME A CHORE.

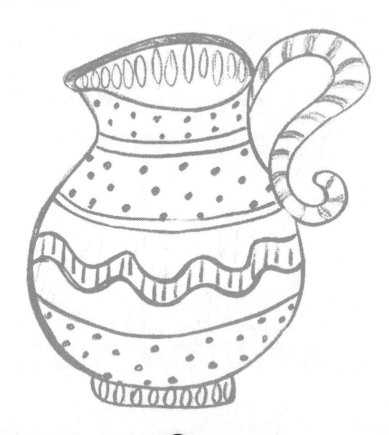

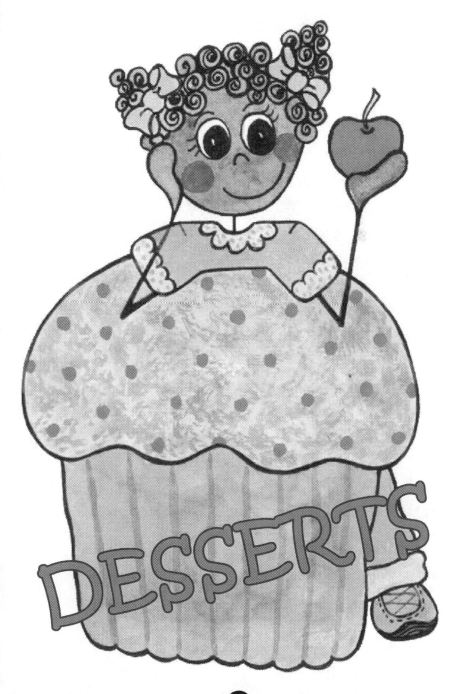

# PRUNE CAKE DELIGHT

1 vanilla cake recipe (see Dessert Basics)
4 Cups heavy cream whipped (see Dessert Basics)
3 Cups raisins
4 Cups seedless prunes
½ Cup raw sugar
1 ½ Cups rum or orange juice

Bake the vanilla cake in two greased and floured 9 inch round cake pans for 25 to 30 minutes or till done (see Dessert Basics). Set aside and cool. Cut each round in half horizontally. Cook the raisins, the prunes, the sugar and the water in a large pot on medium heat for about 5 minutes stirring constantly to prevent sticking. Set aside to cool then blend till pureed. The mixture should be thick. Refrigerate. To assemble first lay one of the halves on a plate or round tray. Spread 1/4 of the prune and raisin mixture on the cake. Spread a cup of the whipped cream over the prune and raisin mixture. Cover with the second layer of cake and repeat the process. Do this with the remaining layers. "Ice" the cake all around with the remaining whipped cream. Use the remaining ¼ of the prune and raisin mixture to drizzle decoratively over the cream on the cake. If mixture is too thick, water it down with some orange juice before drizzling over the cake. Keep cake in the refrigerator and serve cold.


## "3 MILK" DESSERT – ONE WAY

Mix ingredients for one muffin recipe. (see Dessert Basics)
Bake in a 10 inch round or square or an equivalent rectangle pan. Bake as directed. If you are going to use the same pan to prepare the dessert then

leave in pan once you have baked it, if not, remove cake and place in the dish you are going to use. Cut to fit the dish. Of course you can use an oven proof glass dish and then leave the cake in the same dish.

Mix the following 4 ingredients and pour over the baked muffin mixture.

2 Cups cream
2 Cups evaporated milk
2 Cups condensed milk
½ Tsp. grated lemon peel

Now for the topping:
½ Lb. strawberries
1 Cup of strawberry jam or preserves

Wash the strawberries, remove the leaves and slice. In a pot mix the strawberries with the strawberry jam and heat over medium heat till mixture is blended. Cool thoroughly and spread evenly over the milk soaked muffin cake. Refrigerate and serve cold.

Topping the dessert with whipped cream makes it even better.

2 cups of whipped cream (optional)


## "3" MILK DESSERT – MY WAY

1 muffin recipe (see Dessert Basics) and follow instructions)

Bake in an oven proof glass or ceramic 10 x 10 inch square dish or a similar size rectangle. Leave the cake in the pan. Allow cake to cool.

Mix together these three ingredients
1 Can of condensed milk
1 Can of evaporated milk
1 Cup heavy cream

And pour over the cake. Refrigerate till the cream mixture has soaked in and the cake is cold to the touch.

Whisk the following ingredients
¼ Cup heavy cream
¼ Cup condensed milk
¼ Cup evaporated milk
¼ Cup lemon juice

And spread evenly over the top of the dessert. (Do not worry if the mixture curdles when you add the lemon juice). Once you whisk it, it will once again be smooth and creamy. Refrigerate and serve cold.

## "NO BAKE" LEMON PIE

1 Graham cracker pie crust (see Dessert Basics) baked and cooled

2 Cans condensed milk
3 Cups cream cheese
1 Cup lemon juice
½ Tsp. grated lemon rind

Whisk the lemon juice, lemon rind and the condensed milk together. By the way, it helps if all your ingredients are cold before mixing. Whip the cream cheese and fold into the condensed milk mixture. Spoon mixture into your cooled crust. Refrigerate and serve cold.

## BROWNIES

2 Cups all purpose flour
2 Cups raw or brown sugar
 1 Tsp. bicarbonate of soda
¼ Tsp. salt
1 Cup sour cream
½ Cup butter, room temperature

1 Tsp. vanilla
½ Cup water
½ Cup unsweetened dark cocoa powder
1 Cup chopped nuts
1 Cup semi sweet chocolate chunks

In a large bowl mix the cocoa, flour, bicarbonate of soda, salt, sugar, chocolate chunks and the nuts. With a hand held beater or whisk, mix the softened butter and sour cream for ½ a minute then add the water and vanilla beating or whisking for another half a minute. Add the wet ingredients to the dry ingredients and beat with the hand held beater or whisk just enough to mix the ingredients. Do not over beat. Bake in a greased and floured 9×9 inch baking pan in a 175°C (350°F) oven for about 15 minutes. Then turn the oven down to 150°C (300°F) for another 20 to 25 minutes. Check on the brownies. If you want your brownies gooey, the toothpick, when inserted, should come out a little bit chocolaty. If not, leave in the oven a little longer and wait till the toothpick comes out clean. Either way the brownies will be delicious.

## CARROT TORTE

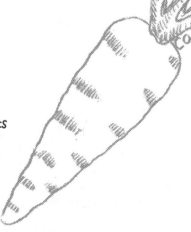

2 Cups flour
1 Cup raw sugar
1 Tsp baking powder
1 Tsp baking soda
3 Cups finely shredded carrot
1 Cup peach yoghurt
1 Cup dried peaches or apricots
2 Tbsp. brandy or rum
½ Cup grape seed or canola oil
1 Tsp. vanilla

Cut the dried peaches or apricots into small pieces. Put them in a microwave safe bowl and add 2 tbsp of rum or brandy. Cover and microwave for 15 seconds. Set aside to cool. Mix the dry ingredients with a whisk. (This is a great tip: A whisk does a great job mixing the dry ingredients evenly and leaves them light and airy which in turn makes for a lighter cake ) Put the apricots into the flour mixture and toss with your fingers making sure that each piece is separated. Mix the carrot, oil, vanilla and peach yoghurt preferably in a processor or by hand till well blended. Now fold the flour mixture into the carrot mixture. Mix well but do not beat. Bake in a 9 inch cheesecake pan in a 175°C (350°F) oven for 40 to 45 minutes. Cool before removing from pan.

## CHEESE AND APPLE TORTE (not a conventional cake as you will see)

2 2/3 Cups flour
1 1/3 Cups raw sugar
4 tsp baking powder
½ tsp baking soda
1 Tbsp. grated orange peel
2/3 Cup milk
2/3 Cup orange juice
1 Tsp. vanilla
½ Cup butter softened
½ Cup plain yoghurt
1 Cup Spanish style white cheese finely grated
1 ½ grated parmesan
2 Cups of sliced apple
1 Tsp. lime juice

Peel, core and slice your apples and toss with the lime juice. Set aside.
Mix your Spanish style white cheese and the grated parmesan. Set aside.

Mix all the dry ingredients thoroughly. Whisk the yoghurt, butter, orange juice, vanilla, grated orange peel. Now mix in the milk.  Mix these wet ingredients with the dry ingredients just till blended.  Do not beat. Put 1/3 of the mixture in the bottom of a greased and floured 10 in. cheesecake pan, previously lined with wax paper, cover with 1/3 of the apple slices and 1/3 of the mixed grated cheeses. Repeat this step with remaining ingredients ending with the apple and grated cheese on top. Bake in 175°C (350°F) oven for about 40 minutes. I recommend testing, with a metal skewer or long toothpick after 30 minutes. As I have mentioned before, **cakes are temperamental.** They could take less or more time depending on the oven or the area where you live (see Dessert Basics). The tester should come out clean when done. **The apple and cheese combination makes this cake different and yummyyy**

## GRANOLA AND COFFEE- COFFEE CAKE

Granola topping
¼ Cup  butter
½ Tsp. cinnamon powder
1 Cup oatmeal
¼ Cup oat bran
¼ Cup wheat germ
½ Cup raw sugar
3 Tbsp. flour
1 Cup chopped nuts

Cake mixture
¼ Tsp. salt
1 ½ Tsp. baking powder
½ Tsp. baking soda
1¾ Cups flour
1/3 Cup raw sugar
¼ Cup sour cream

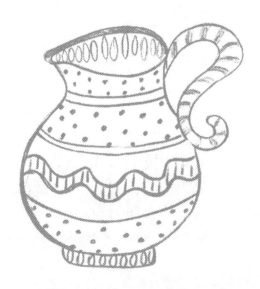

¾ Cup milk
½ Tsp. vanilla
¼ Cup oil (Canola, grape seed or olive oil)

2 Tbsp. Coffee crystals (This is to sprinkle over the batter)

Toss the topping ingredients together till well mixed and the butter is incorporated evenly. Set aside.

Mix the dry ingredients for the cake batter in one bowl and mix the wet ingredients in another bowl. Mix the wet and the dry ingredients together just till evenly blended. Do not over mix. Place half of the batter in a 9x9 inch cake pan. Sprinkle half of the coffee crystals evenly over batter. Repeat with remaining batter and coffee crystals. Top with the mixed granola spreading evenly and patting down gently. Bake in a 150°C (300°F) oven, for about ½ an hour or till tester comes out clean.

## EASY CHOCOLATE FUDGE ICING

1 Can condensed milk
2 Oz. of bitter cooking chocolate
2 Tbsp. butter

Place condensed milk in a double boiler with the chocolate. Stir till chocolate melts (mixture will turn a grayish color). Cook in the double boiler stirring constantly for a couple of minutes. Add the butter and beat thoroughly over heat for about another minute. This can be used as both an icing and a filling. "Easy as pie"

## CHOCOLATE FUDGE CAKE

2 Cups flour
1 ½ Cups raw sugar

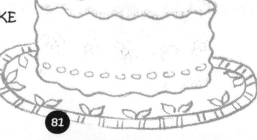

81

½ Cups unsweetened cocoa powder
1 ½ Tsp. baking soda
½ Tsp. Salt
1½ Cups milk
½ Cup yogurt
½ Cup butter
½ Tsp. vanilla

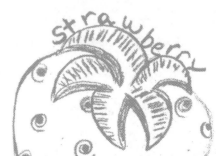

Mix the flour, sugar, baking soda, cocoa powder and salt with the whisk. Whisk or beat together the butter and the yogurt. Now add the milk and the vanilla, a little at a time. Add the wet ingredients all at once to the dry ingredients and beat with the whisk or with the hand held beaters for about a minute. Pour the batter into a 9 inch cheesecake pan, previously lined with wax paper and bake for about 40 minutes in a 175° (350°F) oven. Remember you can test to see if the cake is done by using a skewer or toothpick. If it comes out clean the cake is done.

## STRAWBERRY AND RHUBARB PRESERVE

3 Cups chopped rhubarb
1 Lb. of frozen or fresh strawberries
1 Cup raw sugar

The rhubarb should be washed and peeled before chopping. You can do this with a potato peeler or with a knife. If using fresh strawberries make sure to wash before using and then cut into slices. Cut the rhubarb stalks into small chunks. Put all the ingredients in a pot and bring to a boil over medium heat. Cook till mixture thickens to a spreading consistency. Cool. Store in a clean jar, in the refrigerator. Great to eat on ice cream, on bread or as a cake filling.

## SHERWOOD FORREST CAKE (there are 4 steps to this recipe)

Step 1. - 1 recipe Chocolate Fudge Cake (see recipe)
Step 2. - 1 recipe Rhubarb Preserve (see recipe)
Step 3. - Syrup
¼ Cup rum, brandy or orange liqueur
1 Cup water
1 Cup sugar
Mix the water and the sugar in a pot and cook over medium heat till the mixture resembles, a thin syrup. Add brandy, rum or liqueur
Step 4. - 3 Cups cream, whipped (see Dessert Basics)

When the cake has cooled completely cut horizontally in three. (See Dessert Basics) Place one layer on a plate and pour one third of the syrup over the cake. Spread half of the strawberry and rhubarb preserve on top. Place second layer on top. Repeat the procedure and place the last layer of cake on top. Drizzle the remaining syrup on this layer and proceed to ice the cake with the whipped cream. Refrigerate and serve cold.

If you are wondering if it is worth the effort, it is.

## VEGAN CHOCOLATE CAKE

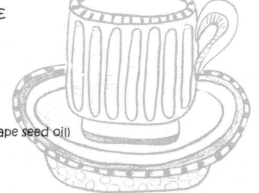

2 ½ Cups flour
1 1/3 Cups sugar
1 Tsp. salt
2 Tsp. baking soda
2/3 Cup cocoa
2/3 Cup oil (Canola, olive or grape seed oil)
1 Tsp. vanilla
1 Tbsp. vinegar
2 ¼ Cups hot water

Mix dry ingredients in a bowl and mix liquids in another bowl. Mix the dry ingredients with the liquids and beat by hand or with a hand held mixer for

1 minute. Do not over beat. Cut a piece of wax paper to fit the bottom of a 10 in. cheesecake pan, pour in the batter and bake in a 175°C or (350°F) oven for about 45 minutes or till the tester comes out clean.

## MY TIRAMISU RECIPE

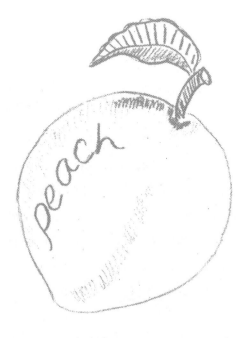

Cake ingredients
2 Cups flour
2/3 Cup sugar
2 Tsp. baking powder
½ Tsp. baking soda
¼ Tsp. salt
1 Cup milk
1/3 Cup butter
1 Tsp. vanilla
¼ Cup plain yogurt

Custard Ingredients
2 Cups milk, room temperature
3 Tbsp. cornstarch
3 Tbsp. raw sugar
3 Tbsp. Kahlua (coffee liqueur)
2 Cups fresh whipping cream, whipped (see Dessert Basics))
8 oz. of Mascarpone Cheese or cream cheese (room temperature)

Coffee syrup ingredients
4 Cups water
½ C sugar
2 Tbsp instant coffee crystals
3 Tbsp. rum
These ingredients are for adding between cake layers and on top
3 Tbsp. cocoa powder
6 Oz. of semi-sweet chocolate, grated

Start by, making a thin syrup. Add the water, sugar and instant coffee and cook at a slow boil for about 20 minutes. Add the rum and set aside to cool.

Now make the custard; Dissolve the cornstarch in the milk and stir in the sugar. Place over medium heat and bring to a boil stirring frequently so that the mixture does not stick or burn. Place a piece of plastic film over the top, patting down carefully. This prevents the custard from forming a skin. Set aside to cool. Whip the cream according to directions in the Dessert Basics section and place in the refrigerator till it is needed. When the custard has cooled thoroughly, fold it in with the whipped cream and the mascarpone or cream cheese. Do not beat but be sure that the ingredients are well blended. Keep in the refrigerator till needed.

To make the cake; Mix the flour, the sugar, baking soda, baking powder and the salt thoroughly with a whisk. Whisk together the milk, butter, yogurt and vanilla and add to the dry ingredients. Blended well but do not beat. Bake in a greased and floured jelly roll pan in a 175°C (350°F) oven for about 20 (give or take) minutes. If you have a Teflon liner or some wax paper to line the bottom of the jellyroll pan it would be even better. Cake should be a nice golden color when done. Cool

Select your dish. Spoon a 1/3 of the coffee syrup in the bottom of the dish then cut half of the cake to fit the dish. **Spoon half** of the remaining liquid over the cake then **spread half** of the cream mixture over this. Place 1 ½ Tbsp. of cocoa in a sieve and dust lightly over cream mixture. Then hold grater over the cake and grate 1/2 of the chocolate evenly over the cocoa. Repeat process by placing another layer of cake over the cream and spooning the remaining syrup over it. Spread remaining cream mixture over the coffee soaked cake. Finish the whole process by lightly dusting the remaining cocoa and grating the rest of the chocolate over the cream. Serve very cold. If your refrigerator is not that cold then place the dessert in the freezer for about 20 to 30 minutes before serving. Trust me, it makes all the difference

## HONEY DRENCHED ORANGE CAKE

Ingredients for syrup
2/3 Cup honey
1 ½ Cups orange juice
3 Tbsp. Orange marmalade (Remove the peel if you prefer)
4 Tbsp. orange liqueur or rum (add a bit more if you want it stronger)
4 Tbsp. Butter

Place all the ingredients in a sauce pot and heat thoroughly (do not boil). Set a ¼ Cup aside. Keep the rest of the syrup in the pot to reheat when ready to use.

Cake ingredients
2 Cups flour
¼ Cup sugar
3 Tsp. baking powder
½ Tsp. baking soda
½ Tsp. salt
1 Tsp. grated orange peel
1 Cup milk
1/3 Cup yogurt
1/3 Cup butter
1 Tsp. orange essence
2 Tbsp. finely chopped crystallized orange peel

Whisk together the flour, baking powder, baking soda and salt. Whisk the butter with the sugar for 1 minute then add the yogurt and the milk. Fold in the dry ingredients with the grated and crystallized orange peel.

Grease and flour a 9inx9in cake pan. Cut a piece of wax paper the size of your baking pan and place it in the bottom. Pour batter in and bake in a 175°C (350°F) oven for 25 to 30 minutes or till golden and the tester comes out clean.

While the cake is still in the pan poke some holes in the top with a fork. Spoon the remaining hot syrup evenly over the cake. (Do not use the ¼ Cup of syrup previously set aside). Allow to soak for about 5 minutes then turn cake over onto a plate.

For the topping

1 or 1 ½ Cups sliced almonds

¼ Cup reserved syrup

Place the sliced almonds on a tray and bake in a 150°C (300°F) oven till golden in color. Keep a watchful eye so that they do not burn. Toss the almonds with the ¼ Cup of reserved syrup and spread evenly over the cake. As an added idea you could cut the cake into squares and serve each square in a pretty cupcake liner.

## CHOCOLATE CHIP COOKIES

1 ¼ Cups of flour
1/3 Cup oatmeal
1 Tbsp. wheat germ
½ Tsp. salt
½ Tsp. baking soda
½ Cup raw sugar
1/3 Cup soy or regular milk
½ Cup butter
1 Tsp. vanilla
1 Cup chocolate chunks, sweet or semi sweet
½ Cup chopped nuts (your choice)

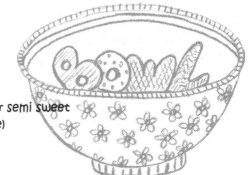

Mix the flour, salt, baking soda, oatmeal and wheat germ together. Whisk or beat the sugar with the butter till creamy and add the soy or regular milk and vanilla. Mix thoroughly and then add the dry ingredients. Whisk or beat till blended. Fold in the chocolate chunks and the nuts. Grease cookie sheet. Measure the batter with a teaspoon. Leave space for them to spread. Bake in a 150°C (300°F) oven for about 15 to 20 minutes. They should be a nice golden color. (See cookie tips in Dessert Basics)

## "WOULD YOU BELIEVE" EGGLESS CHEESECAKE

I made my hubby and myself very happy when I came up with recipe. Honest

1 Graham cracker crust recipe (see Desert Basics section)

### FILLING:
24 oz of Cream Cheese (3, 8oz packages) room temperature
1 Cup sugar
1 Tsp. vanilla
½ Tsp. of shredded lemon or orange peel (optional)
¼ Cup sour cream
3 Tbsp. flour
2 Tbsp. arrowroot
1 Tbsp. milk

Dissolve arrowroot with the milk and sour cream. Now beat this mixture with the cream cheese, sugar, orange or lemon peel and vanilla for about a minute. (Note: You can add any other flavoring you prefer instead of the vanilla.) Pour into the unbaked graham crust. Bake in a 175°C (350°F) for about 30 minutes. You must watch carefully so that the mixture does not start bubbling. If you notice this happening, remove from oven immediately. Cool and then refrigerate.

You will enjoy the cheesecake as is. Or you can: 1. Top with a store bought cherry pie filling, for instance, Or 2. Heat a jar of strawberry fruit preserves in a pot and add a cup of sliced fresh strawberries. Stir till thoroughly mixed and heated through. Spread mixture over the cooled cheesecake. Serve cold.

## BUMPY ROAD GRANOLA COOKIES

½ Cup butter
½ Cup raw sugar or brown sugar
4 Tbsp of milk
1 Tbsp molasses
1 ½ Cups flour
½ Tsp. baking soda
¼ Tsp. salt
½ Tsp. cinnamon
½ Tsp. ground cloves
½ Tsp. nutmeg
1 Cup rolled oats
2 Tbsp wheat bran
1 Tbsp wheat germ
½ Cup of nuts (your choice) roughly chopped
1 Cup crystallized fruit, raisins, sultanas or currants (a mixture is great)

Mix the flour, wheat germ, wheat bran, cinnamon, nutmeg, ground cloves, salt and baking soda. Beat the butter, molasses and the sugar for about a minute then add ½ the flour and mix. Add the milk and oatmeal and mix. Add the remaining flour. Add the fruit and the nuts and mix. Grease cookie sheet. Measure out the cookies with a teaspoon or tablespoon. Flatten each cookie with your hand or with a fork. Leave space between each cookie for them to spread. Bake in a 150°C (300°F) oven for about 15 to 20 minutes. Cookies should be golden in color and crunchy when cooled. Cookies are always fun. Store in a tightly sealed jar.

## CITRUS TEA COOKIES

½ Cup butter, softened
2 Tsp. orange zest
½ Tsp. lemon zest
½ Tsp. tangerine zest
½ Cup plus 1 tbsp milk
1 ¾ Cups flour
½ Tsp. salt
½ Tsp. baking soda
1 Cup raw sugar
1 Tsp. orange or lemon essence

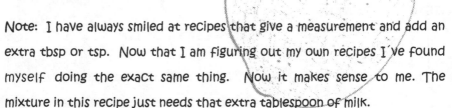

Note: I have always smiled at recipes that give a measurement and add an extra tbsp or tsp. Now that I am figuring out my own recipes I've found myself doing the exact same thing. Now it makes sense to me. The mixture in this recipe just needs that extra tablespoon of milk.

Mix the flour, salt, baking soda and the orange, lemon and tangerine zest together. Beat the butter with the sugar till creamy. Add the essence and half the milk. Stir (so that you don't splatter yourself) then mix well. Add half the flour mixture and beat till blended. Repeat the procedure with the remaining milk and flour. On a greased or non-stick cookie sheet spoon a teaspoon or tablespoon of the batter for each cookie. Leave space between cookies to make room for spreading. Bake in a 175°C (350°F) oven for 15 minutes or till edges are golden. The cookies are crispy when cool. Keep in an air tight container. See Dessert Basics for cookie tips.

## GINGER COOKIES

2 ¼ Cup flour
½ Tsp. salt
½ to 1 Cup brown sugar or raw sugar Note: I use only ½ a cup of sugar because I prefer the cookies less sweet. Adjust sugar to your taste.
¾ Cup butter, softened
¼ Cup molasses
1 Tbsp. honey
1 Tsp. baking soda
1 Tsp. Ginger
1 Tsp. cinnamon
½ Tsp. ground cloves

Beat the softened butter and the sugar for about a minute till creamy. Add the molasses and the honey and mix well. Mix the flour, salt, cinnamon, ginger, cloves, baking soda and salt. Add the flour mixture to the butter mixture and beat till thoroughly combined. Bake the cookies on a greased cookie sheet in a 175°C (350°F) oven for 10 minutes. If you like them really crispy then leave for another couple of minutes but just be careful not to let them burn. I use a teaspoon (or tablespoon for a bigger cookie) for each cookie and then use a fork to press down till you have a ¼ of an inch disk. You can also measure out each cookie and make a ball and roll the ball in some sugar then bake as indicated above. This will, of course, make the cookies sweeter.

## PASSION FRUIT DELIGHT

First step.
8 Cups of plain yoghurt
3 Tbsp. sugar

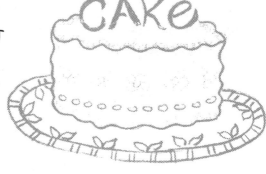

The day before you make this dessert, you must line a large strainer with coffee filters and place the strainer over a bowl. Now mix the yoghurt and the sugar and pour it into the coffee filter lined strainer. Place in the refrigerator and drain till yoghurt becomes very thick. You will probably have about 4 cups of thick yoghurt left. Keep refrigerated till needed.

For the cake:

2 2/3 Cups flour
2/3 Cup raw sugar
4 Tsp. baking powder
½ Tsp. baking soda
1 1/3 Cup milk
½ Cup butter, softened
½ Cup plain yoghurt
2 Tsp. vanilla
1 Tsp. vinegar

Grease and flour a 10 inch cake pan. Mix the dry ingredients and set aside. Beat the butter for a second then add the vanilla and the vinegar stirring first then beating for half a minute or so. Mix the yoghurt and the milk and add to the butter mixture and beat for about half a minute more. Add the dry ingredients and beat at low speed just till the ingredients are evenly mixed, approximately, half a minute. Your batter will sponge up so pour in the prepared cake pan right away (before the spongy effect goes) and bake in a preheated oven 175°C (350°F) for about 40 minutes or till it is a nice golden brown and the tester comes out clean.

To make the passion fruit syrup:

1 ½ Cups sugar
1 ½ Cups water

In a pot, mix and boil the sugar and the water, over medium heat (a slow boil) for 8 minutes. Add 1 ½ Cup of concentrated passion fruit juice to the syrup and stir till well blended. Set aside.

When the cake has cooled thoroughly place it in the freezer till it is firm enough to cut into three layers. Put your first layer on you cake plate and pour 1/3 of your syrup over it. Spread 1/3 of the yogurt over the soaked cake and place the second layer of cake over this. Repeat process with remaining layers. The last syrup drenched layer will be covered with the remaining 1/3 portion of yogurt. Keep in the refrigerator and serve cold. This cake is very refreshing.

## COCONUT PIE

2 Packages of vanilla pudding
1 Cup coconut milk
2 Cups milk
2 Cups of whipped cream
1 Cup dehydrated coconut, grated
2 Tsp. coconut essence
½ Tsp. vanilla (optional)
One 10 inch pie pastry shell (see Dessert Basics section for pastry recipe)

Prepare pie pastry and bake. Set aside and cool.

Pie Filling

My pudding instructions call for 4 cups of milk so if I use two pudding mixes I will only use 2 cups of milk and 1 cup of coconut milk. I am eliminating 1 cup of liquid. This is because I want my filling to have a thicker consistency. (Note: Quantities may vary according to package instructions. Always use less liquid) Mix the contents of the package with the milk, coconut milk and coconut essence. Cook over medium heat till mixture bubbles and thickens. Let boil for about a minute stirring constantly so that the mixture does not stick to the bottom of the pot. Place a piece of plastic film over the top of the pudding. This is to prevent a skin forming over the top of the pudding. Cool and then refrigerate. Meanwhile whip the cream (see Dessert Basics section on whipping cream) and refrigerate. Put the coconut on a cookie sheet and bake in a 150°C (300°F) oven till golden in color. Stir a couple of times so that you get an even color. Set aside to cool. Fold the whipped cream into the cooled coconut pudding then spoon the mixture into the cooled pie shell. Cover the top with the grated coconut and refrigerate. Keep really cold.

P.S. Do not let the instructions scare you off. The pie is worth it.

## LEMON PIE "CHEESECAKE" (It is done in a jiffy!)

3 package of 8 Oz. of cream cheese
1 1/3 Cups condensed milk
1 Cup milk
4 Tbsp. Cornstarch
½ Cup plus 1 Tbsp lemon juice
1 recipe graham cracker crust (see dessert basics section)

Prepare crust and bake according to recipe. Cool.

Mix milk and cornstarch and cook over medium heat till the mixture bubbles and thickens. Note: If the milk and cornstarch cook up lumpy, strain before mixing with the other ingredients. Mix the lemon juice with the condensed milk. It will thicken automatically. Now add the cooked cornstarch mixture and cream cheese and mix till thoroughly blended. Pour into the cooled graham cracker crust. Refrigerate and serve cold.

Here are some more muffin recipes that I hope you enjoy. I like making **muffins because they usually always go well. Vegans or the lactose intolerant can omit the cheese and replace the butter for oil in the following recipes.** See Dessert Basics for tips on making muffins.

## ORANGE PEEL MUFFINS (WITHOUT THE CRUMB TOPPING THEY ARE VEGANS WORTHY)

1 Cup flour
½ Cup soy flour
¼ Cup wheat bran
1 Tbsp. wheat germ
½ Tsp. salt
½ Tsp. baking soda
2 Tsp. baking powder
1/3 Cup sugar
¼ Cup finely chopped candied orange peel (optional-it is not necessary but it sure is a great touch)
¼ Cup olive oil
½ Cup soy milk
½ Cup orange juice
1 Tsp. orange essence (optional)

Crumb topping
½ Cup flour
½ Cup brown sugar
2 tbsp butter
¼ Cup chopped nuts

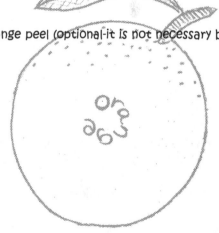

Mix dry ingredients in a bowl and stir with a wire whisk. Add the orange peel to the flour mixture and stir till coated. Mix the wet ingredients and whip, just for a second, with a wire whisk. Mix the wet and the dry ingredients together just till blended. Do not beat. Do not worry if the mixture looks lumpy.

Mix the crumb topping ingredients with your fingers till it resembles coarse crumbs. Add the chopped nuts and mix.

Fill the greased muffin cups about 2/3 full and sprinkle the topping over the top of each muffin. Bake in a 200°C (400°F) oven for 12 minutes or till done. Remember to add a little water to any empty muffin cup.

## BRUNCH MUFFINS (TO BE VEGAN WORTHY JUST OMIT THE CHEESE)

1¾ Cups flour
2 Tsp. smoked paprika
¼ Tsp. powdered turmeric
½ Tsp. salt
Freshly ground Black pepper
1 Tbsp. sugar
2 Tsp. baking powder
½ Tsp. baking soda
¾ Cup beer
¼ Cup extra virgin olive oil or grape seed oil
1/3 Cup finely chopped green bell pepper
1/3 Cup finely chopped red bell pepper
¼ Cup finely chopped shallots
1 Cup of grated cheddar cheese

Preheat the oven 200°C (400°F). Grease medium size muffin pans. Thoroughly mix the flour, salt, smoked paprika, baking soda, baking powder, freshly ground black pepper, the cheese and the sugar. Mix in the chopped red and green bell pepper and the chopped onion till evenly distributed in the flour. In another bowl whisk together the oil and the beer and pour it in with the flour and veggie mixture. Do not beat, just fold in the ingredients. Fill the muffin pans ¾ full and bake 15 to 25 minutes or till done. They should be a nice golden color. Some muffins take less time but these have all the veggies so I like to make sure that they get cooked. This will just fill 10 of the medium size muffin pan. Fill empty muffin cups with a little water. See Dessert Basics for muffin tips.

## CARROT MUFFINS (ALSO A VEGAN RECIPE)

1 ¾ Cups flour
2 Tbsp. wheat bran
1 Tbsp. wheat germ
2 Tsp. baking powder
2 Tbsp. brown sugar
½ Tsp. salt
¼ Tsp. powdered turmeric
1 Cup grated carrot
2 Tbsp. molasses
½ Cup Pony Malta (a sweet malt carbonated beverage) or root beer
¼ Cup extra virgin olive oil
For the topping
1/3 Cup roughly chopped walnuts
¼ Cup sugar

Mix the flour, sugar, wheat germ, wheat bran, turmeric, salt, sugar and baking powder. Stir the oil, molasses and Pony Malta or root beer together with the grated carrot. Fold this mixture into the dry ingredients but do not beat. Fill grease muffin pans ¾ full (only 10) and top with a few chopped nuts and a sprinkling of sugar. Bake in a 200°C (400° F) oven for 15 to 20 minutes. As always, keep an eye on them.  See Dessert Basics for tips.


## GRANOLA MUFFINS (ALSO VEGAN WORTHY)

1 ¾ Cup flour
1 Tbsp. wheat germ
1 Tbsp. wheat bran
1/3 Cup raw sugar
2 Tsp. baking powder
½ Tsp. salt
1 Tsp. vinegar
1 Cup Soy milk
¼ Cup olive oil
½ Cup of dried fruit (cranberries, cherries, blueberries etc.)
½ Cup chopped nuts of choice
½ Cup raisins

Topping:
1/2 Cup finely chopped nuts
2 Tbsp. brown sugar
½ Tsp. cinnamon
Mix together.

In a mixing bowl combine flour, sugar, baking powder, salt, wheat germ and wheat bran. Toss in the raisins, nuts and dried fruit till coated. In a small mixing bowl whisk together the milk and vinegar and add to the dry ingredients and stir just till moistened (will look lumpy, no problem). Fill greased muffin pan ¾ full and top with a sprinkling of the topping. Bake in a preheated 200°C (400°F) oven for about 15 minutes or a little more.  Use the tester to see if they need a little more time. Better safe than sorry.

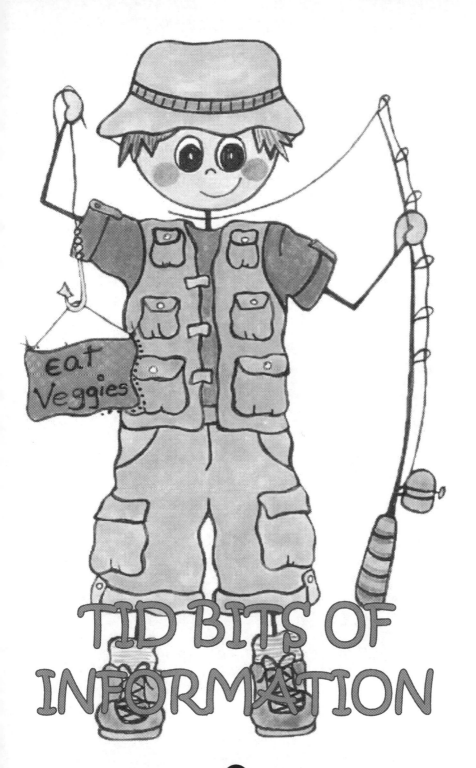

TID BITS OF INFORMATION

## TURMERIC POWDER

My savory dishes are usually laced with turmeric not only for its flavor but for its medicinal purposes. Turmeric (*Curcuma longa*) is a rhizomatous herbaceous perennial plant of the ginger family (Zingiberaceae). It is native to tropical South Asia. It is usually presented to us in powder form which comes from the root. Most importantly it is medicinal. Usually found in Indian food but I use it just about in every recipe. I add ½ a teaspoonful which, as far as I am concerned, does not really alter the flavor of what ever savory dish I am preparing. Why, most would ask? Well it helps whenever you have an inflammation problem. It is specially recommended for prostate inconveniences. I do not suppose that this has been scientifically proven but my hubby says it works so I use it in everything I can. As far as I know it does no harm but nevertheless consult your doctor. It tastes good and has a lovely yellow color.

## GINGER, TURMERIC, LIME, GREEN TEA AND HONEY WATER

½ Cup grated ginger root
4 lemons
¾ Tsp. turmeric powder
¼ Cup honey
3 Green tea bags or 2 Tbsp. lose green tea
6 Cups water

Steep the tea in hot water. Bring 2 cups of water to a boil with the turmeric and add the grated ginger root. Ps: You do not have to peel the root. Just wash and grate. Remove from heat and steep for 15 minutes. Strain the green tea and the turmeric and ginger water and pour into a jug. Preferably a glass or stainless steel jug since the turmeric will stain the plastic jug. Add the honey and the juice from the lemons stirring well. Fill jug with the remaining water. Keep refrigerated. It is both refreshing and medicinal

## LINSEED

Flax seed or linseed is very good for everyone but specially, for vegetarians. It is a way of obtaining omega-3, 6 and 9. It can act as a laxative so you must be careful and as always you should consult your doctor before consuming. It is best to have the seed and grind it yourself just before you drink it. Once ground, it begins to oxidize and lose its medicinal properties. A coffee grinder will do the job but if you do not have one then soak the seed in a glass of water for about 15 to 20 minutes and then put it in the blender and blend till nicely ground.

## COFFEE GRINDER

Coffee grinders are more than just a coffee grinder. If you get one on sale it is good to have an extra one to use for grinding spices, flax seed and other types of seeds and even pepper corns. This way it won't ruin the flavor of your coffee.

## COFFEE FILTERS

Paper coffee filters are super useful. For instance, they are great for straining yoghurt. Put the yoghurt in the strainer and leave in the refrigerator for a couple of hours and it is ready for using as a topping for pancakes or a healthy icing on a cupcake or for mixing in a recipe. The paper coffee filter is hygienic since you throw it away after each use.

# HOW TO MAKE GLUTEN

In this cookbook you will see "Gluten" and "Tofu" in the recipes so I think is only normal that I include the recipes to make them. I warn you, they are kind of tedious to make but if you are industrious it is not a problem. I will be honest, however, I have never made it and I don't think I ever will. I prefer to buy it.

4 lbs flour (not cake flour)
Water

Put the flour in a large bowl, add water and knead till you remove all the lumps and the dough is nice and smooth. Cover the dough with water and leave submerged for half and hour. Now you must rinse the dough over and over, changing the water as the starch from the flour comes out and turns the water cloudy. Continue this process until the water comes out clean. You will be left with only the protein of the flour. Dough should be smooth but not sticky. Strain the liquid so that you do not loose any of the little pieces of dough. Set aside while you prepare for the next step.

5 cloves of garlic
2 large red onions
1 large red bell pepper
1 Cup chopped spring onion
1 vegetable cube
1 Tsp. ground thyme
1 Tsp. ground bay leaf
1 tsp. ground coriander
2 Tbsp. oil

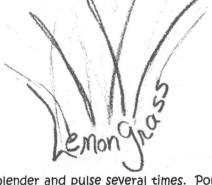

Lemon Grass

Place all the above ingredients in a blender and pulse several times. Pour this mixture over the dough. Knead the dough till the mixture blends in thoroughly. Place the seasoned dough into a large pot of water and boil for an hour. Leave in the water till cool. It is ready to slice and dice.

## HOW TO MAKE SOY MILK AND TOFU

1 Lb. of soy bean
1 Tsp. Epson salt
2 Tbsp. lime juice
Water
Cheese cloth and string

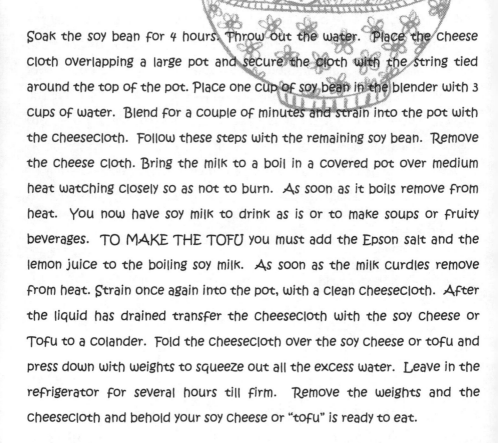

Soak the soy bean for 4 hours. Throw out the water. Place the cheese cloth overlapping a large pot and secure the cloth with the string tied around the top of the pot. Place one cup of soy bean in the blender with 3 cups of water. Blend for a couple of minutes and strain into the pot with the cheesecloth. Follow these steps with the remaining soy bean. Remove the cheese cloth. Bring the milk to a boil in a covered pot over medium heat watching closely so as not to burn. As soon as it boils remove from heat. You now have soy milk to drink as is or to make soups or fruity beverages. TO MAKE THE TOFU you must add the Epson salt and the lemon juice to the boiling soy milk. As soon as the milk curdles remove from heat. Strain once again into the pot, with a clean cheesecloth. After the liquid has drained transfer the cheesecloth with the soy cheese or Tofu to a colander. Fold the cheesecloth over the soy cheese or tofu and press down with weights to squeeze out all the excess water. Leave in the refrigerator for several hours till firm. Remove the weights and the cheesecloth and behold your soy cheese or "tofu" is ready to eat.

## ON ANOTHER NOTE

The following is not a cooking recipe but more like a "feel better" recipe. In all honesty I cannot say that it has magical powers but if said from the heart and with gratitude it cannot but have positive results. As in any of my recipes feel free to make your own personal adjustments, customize it if you will. Basically, everyday we should express our thanks for everything good and positive in our personal life and in the lives of our families. This is my personal pep talk and I would like to share it with you.

My home and my family are blessed.
We live in peace and harmony and the Universe protects us.
We are happy and healthy of body and mind and
We are, spiritually and financially wealthy.
We are conscious that we should always be:
Charitable, honest, kind and fair to ourselves and to all living things.

THANK YOU

THANK YOU

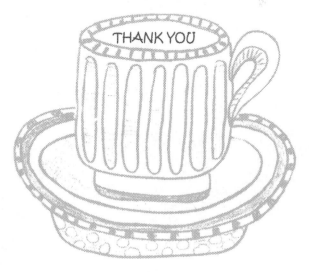

THANK YOU

# GENERAL INDEX

# Notes: